S0-EDI-323

The Neurobiology of Learning

of Learning

Perspectives From
Second Language Acquisition

The Neurobiology of Learning

Perspectives From Second Language Acquisition

John H. Schumann
University of California at Los Angeles

Sheila E. Crowell
University of Washington, Seattle

Nancy E. Jones
University of California at Los Angeles

Namhee Lee
University of California at Riverside

Sara Ann Schuchert
Mid-Wilshire Christian Schools, Los Angeles

Lee Alexandra Wood
STARR Litigation Services, Des Moines, Iowa

LAWRENCE ERLBAUM ASSOCIATES, PUBLISHERS
2004   Mahwah, New Jersey   London

Copyright © 2004 by Lawrence Erlbaum Associates, Inc.
All rights reserved. No part of this book may be repro-
duced in any form, by photostat, microfilm, retrieval system, or any other means, without prior written permission
of the publisher.

Lawrence Erlbaum Associates, Inc., Publishers
10 Industrial Avenue
Mahwah, NJ 07430

Cover design by Kathryn Houghtaling Lacey

Library of Congress Cataloging-in-Publication Data

The neurobiology of learning : perspectives from second language acquisition / John H. Schumann ... [et al.]
　　　　p. cm.
Includes bibliographical references and index.
ISBN 0-8058-4717-0 (alk. paper)

QP408.N495 2004
612.8'233—dc22　　　　　　　　　　2003060656
　　　　　　　　　　　　　　　　　　　　CIP

Books published by Lawrence Erlbaum Associates are printed
on acid-free paper, and their bindings are chosen for strength
and durability.

Printed in the United States of America
10　9　8　7　6　5　4　3　2　1

To Arnold Scheibel

In the early 1980s, Bob Jacobs, then a graduate student in Applied Linguistics at UCLA, began to take neuroscience courses at the Brain Research Institute. There he studied neuroanatomy with Dr. Arnold Scheibel and became both a TA for Dr. Scheibel's classes and an RA in his laboratory. In the 1985–86 academic year when Dr. Wolfgang Klein from the Max Plank Psycholinguistic Institute was a visiting professor at UCLA, Bob arranged for us to meet with Dr. Scheibel on a regular basis to discuss issues of brain and language. As a result of these discussions, Dr. Scheibel offered to teach neuroanatomy to students in Applied Linguistics. The first course was taught in the fall 1987, and it began a long exciting relationship between our Applied Linguistics students and Dr. Scheibel. Applied Linguistics students have been taking neuroanatomy with Dr. Scheibel every other year since then.

Dr. Scheibel is a dynamic teacher who loves his subject. His lectures are like watching Nova three times a week. Learning neuroanatomy is no easy task. A friend, who is an oncological surgeon, recalls his neuroanatomy studies in medical school as similar "to memorizing Amtrak schedules." Indeed a good deal of memorization is necessary, but Dr. Scheibel makes sure we see the brain from multiple perspectives: by dissecting sheep brains, human brains, and working through diagrams in brain atlases, The Human Brain Coloring Book, and in computer visualizations of the substrate.

Slowly but surely the students become comfortable navigating the neural landscape, and then a whole new world opens. They learn about the brain and they learn a science. When humanities students become proficient in a science, it is very empowering—particularly in neuroscience which provides a biological basis for all human activity and which frequently leads to interest in evolution, genetics, and complexity.

Successfully learning neuroscience requires distributed cognition, and it couldn't be done without Dr. Scheibel's generous help beyond the neuroanatomy class. He has served on many of our Applied Linguistics MA thesis committees, PhD qualifying paper committees and PhD dissertation committees. He puts us in touch with other neuroscientists with expertise in our areas of interest. Dr. Scheibel also organizes a monthly meeting of individuals interested in the neurobiology of higher cognitive function. The group has been meeting for about 15 years. When students have finished the neuroanatomy class, they are welcome to join the group and to explore with other neuroscientists a wide range of issues involving brain function.

It is the relationship with Dr. Scheibel that allowed us to write this book. He guided us to the knowledge of neurobiology that we use here to understand SLA, and he has been tolerant and supportive of our linguistic speculations that go beyond the neural data. However, while our inspiration and guidance are his gifts to us, any mistakes are ours.

It is to this wonderful scholar, teacher, gentleman, and friend that we dedicate this book.

Contents

Foreword

There has been a tendency in language acquisition circles to dismiss neuroscience because, as the claim goes, supposedly not enough is known about the brain to make significant contributions to our understanding of how language is acquired. Unfortunately, such claims often reflect an overriding ignorance of underlying neural mechanisms—a dismissive attitude about the neurosciences that must end. This book constitutes a timely contribution to the existing literature by presenting a relatively comprehensive, neurobiological account of certain aspects of second language acquisition. Moreover, the present volume avoids the corticocentric bias that characterizes many brain-language publications—both cortical and subcortical structures receive their appropriate attention here. The chapters in this volume demonstrate, without any apology, that enough is presently known about the brain to inform our conceptualizations of how humans acquire second languages. It thus provides a refreshingly novel, highly integrative contribution to the (second) language acquisition literature.

Historically, the language acquisition mirror, as it were, has reflected behavior back into the "black box" of theoretical mechanisms with little concern for the neurobiological plausibility of those mechanisms. The acquisition literature is replete with such supposed mental mechanisms (e.g., buffers, filters, organizers, Language Acquisition Device, Universal Grammar). Although such cognitive metaphors may help researchers *describe* acquisition at a phenomenological level, they are ultimately of limited *explanatory* value without an underlying neural foundation. With this book, the perspective comes full circle: we are now looking out from the brain itself, letting the neurobiology itself indicate potential signposts along the road of second language acquisition. Such an approach is not for the neurobiologically timid, however, as it requires one to learn the language of the brain for effective academic discourse. It is a long, complex, but intellectually stimulating neural pathway.

Indeed, the impulse for this speculative account of language acquisition began nearly four decades ago with Lenneberg's (1967) landmark publication of *Biological Foundations of Language*, which helped set the general stage for this kind of interdisciplinary undertaking. Within the field of second language acquisition, the major impetus for the neural perspective was provided by the seminal neurofunctional contributions of Lamendella (1977), who claimed that "observation of overt behavior in itself cannot be an adequate basis for understanding the organization of the internal systems that produce behavior" (p. 160). Supplementing Lamendella's functional emphasis, Jacobs (1988) focused more on the underlying neuroanatomical substrate itself, questioning the neural plausibility of linguistic concepts such as Universal Grammar. Finally, the foundation for the current volume developed with a series of subsequent publications by Schumann and his colleagues (Jacobs & Schumann, 1992; Schumann, 1994, 1997; Pulvermüller, 1992; Pulvermüller & Schumann, 1994). Although each of these authors approached the neural underpinnings of language from a slightly different perspective, all had the unwavering conviction that language acquisition researchers need to incorporate a degree of neuroscientific reality into their perceptions of the language acquisition process. Although this neural emphasis is not without its detractors (cf. Eubank & Gregg, 1995), there is no denying the significant advances of recent neuroscientific investigations relative to language acquisition, many of which are discussed in the current volume.

The details in this volume will invariably be modified with future research, but the fundamental insights presented here should guide second language acquisition researchers for years to come. This is very much a work in progress, a work that could only have been realized within an atmosphere inherently supportive of truly interdisciplinary undertakings, such as the UCLA Applied Linguistics and TESL Department, which has led the field of applied linguistics for more than thirty years. More specifically, the Neurobiology of Language Research Group responsible for this volume could not have flourished without the continued, unparalleled guidance of two scholars: John Schumann and Arnold B. Scheibel. They provided the neural underpinnings of this volume, the glia of productive collaboration. It is my sincere hope that this book will further promote such interdisciplinary undertakings by a new generation of neurobiologically knowledgeable investigators.

Bob Jacobs, PhD
Laboratory of Quantitative Neuromorphology
Department of Psychology
The Colorado College
14 East Cache La Poudre
Colorado Springs, CO 80903
USA

Preface

At a colloquium on the Neural Biology of Learning held during the 2002 Conference of the American Association for Applied Linguistics, Nick Ellis pointed out the need to draw more links between the neurobiological mechanisms and second language acquisition. This, of course, is the goal of the research program proposed here. However, it must be noted that constraining links to actual neural mechanisms results in fewer degrees of freedom than inferring acquisition and processes mechanisms from behavior. This is because the "behavior to mechanism" approach allows the imaginative invention of mechanisms that fit that data but that are not necessarily neurobiologically plausible. Schumann (1990) examined five cognitive models in an effort to offer a cognitive account of the Pidginization/Acculturation Model. All five models fit. The cognitive models were neither specific enough nor consistent enough to yield a preference. The brain, on the other hand, anchors mechanisms in actual material, and we know this material is this source of the cognition involved in SLA. Middle level psycholinguistic, neurolinguistic, and cognitive accounts are, of course, extremely helpful. One can't just probe around in the neural tissue looking for learning mechanisms. Psychological theories focus research. But to be productive the psychological models must be answerable to their neuroanatomy and neurophysiology. Given these considerations, we probably have to recognize that developing links between neural mechanisms and SLA may be more difficult, but we believe that this is more than compensated for by the knowledge that the brain is the ultimate mechanism subserving the acquisition of knowledge and skill, and therefore, it is where we should be looking.

The point of this book is not to apply findings in psycholinguistics, neurolinguistics and cognitive studies of language to SLA but rather to promote a neurobiology of language that starts with the brain and moves to behavior. We do not believe the mechanisms we propose are the final word on the issue. We envision a research program that gets modified and expanded as more and more is learned about the brain. We expect that debates will be generated by neurobiologically oriented researchers in SLA about what anatomical and physiological mechanisms are the best candidates to subtend language acquisition. It may be difficult or, even for a long period of time, impossible to test the proposals this research generates. Because of the complexity of the brain and the limitations of current noninvasive imaging technology, empirical research on the hypothesized mechanisms may be some time off. But enough is now known about the brain that it is time to attempt to constrain our theorizing about learning and processing mechanisms by knowledge of the brain. The cognitive tools that have been proposed so far (such as nodes, analyzers, buffers, schemas, filters, operating principles, learning strategies, monitors, and processes such as fossilization, defossilization, pidginization, monitoring, noticing) must have neural correlates, and it is time for the field to attempt to specify them.

For several reasons, we have decided not to simplify the neurobiological information we provide. At a certain level of an abstraction (e.g., that supplied in neurobiology discussions in *The Science Times*), what we say is manifestly true. For example, the hippocampus is involved in declarative memory; the basal ganglia subserves procedural memory. But accounts at this level really explain nothing, and they tend to end discussion rather than opening it up. We see the debate to be in the details—circuits within these areas, circuits among them, local and global physiology, and so on. We envision a field in which these issues are debated with research evidence brought to bear from both language acquisition and neuroscience. As students of SLA become more knowledgeable about the neural substrate, such debates will ensue. But will SLA adopt a biological perspective? We would hope so. SLA is about learning; learning is mediated by the brain. Therefore, neurobiology is as central as linguistics to our enterprise. Additionally, information about the brain is expanding exponentially. Each year at the meeting of the Society for Neuroscience, between 8 and 10,000 presentations are made. A good many of these are directly relevant to learning, and many others provide information that is indirectly relevant: neural development (re, critical periods), motor systems (re, the organization of cognition and articulation), vision (re, reading), prefrontal systems (re, planning, descending control), and so forth. For SLA to ignore this information is to deliberately impose a handicap on its endeavors. But because doing SLA research from the neurobiological perspective requires an investment—one must learn some neurobiology—each researcher has to decide whether overcoming the handicap is worth the investment. The investment is basically a course in neuroanatomy and one in the cell biology of learning and memory. These are available in departments of neuroscience or medicine and will become more generally available to applied linguistics programs as the authors of this book and their followers receive their degrees and become university professors. There was a time when SLA itself was an innovation in the applied linguistics scene. Before the early 1970s, the major expertise expected of professors in Teaching English as a Second Language programs (the precursors of applied linguistics programs) was in linguistics and language teaching methodology. Then departments began hiring faculty because of their expertise in SLA, and courses in this area became wide spread. Because knowledge of the structure and function of the brain is directly relevant to linguistics, teaching, and learning, we would not be surprised if neurobiological training became common in the curricula of applied linguistics, second language acquisition, TESL, and foreign language education programs.

This book constitutes the collaborative efforts of members of the Neurobiology of Language Research Group in the Applied Linguistics and TESL Department at UCLA. Members of this group are trained in neurobiology and then use this knowledge to develop biological accounts of various aspects of applied linguistics. The chapters that comprise this volume were originally written as academic papers—MA theses and PhD qualifying papers. Before the students began these projects, we decided to prepare them as components in what would be a book on the neurobiology of learning. This is that book.

John H. Schumann

Introduction

John H. Schumann

In a seminal paper in second language acquisition, Long (1990) argued that any theory of second language requires the specification of a mechanism to account for the acquisition and development of second language (L2) knowledge and skills. This book is about just such mechanism(s). Like all research on language acquisition and processing mechanisms, this book contains much speculation. Traditional psycholinguistic, neurolinguistic, and cognitive approaches to second language acquisition (SLA) operate by observing linguistic behavior in experimental, clinical, or naturalistic settings, and based on patterns in those data, mechanisms are inferred. These inferences are speculations. Additionally, they are generally abstract characterizations of learner behavior. But to the extent that they actually specify what goes on in the learner's mind/brain, they remain speculations. However, speculation from behavior to mechanism is so standard, ubiquitous and expected in psycholinguistic, neurolinguistic, and cognitive studies that it is frequently unnoticed. Thus, if research procedures and methods of data analysis raise no objections, then the speculations from behavior to mechanism are seen as reasonable and appropriate. However, in this book, we work in the opposite direction. On the basis of well-researched neural mechanisms for motivation, procedural memory, declarative memory, memory consolidation, and attention, we speculate about what language learning behavior could be subserved by these mechanisms. Figure 1 illustrates the difference.

In this book, we explain learning on the basis of domain-general neural mechanisms. Much language acquisition research, particularly in SLA, has followed traditional linguistics in postulating a domain-specific mechanism, a Language Acquisition Device (LAD) or a Universal Grammar (UG). However, after several decades of research within this paradigm, is not clear that UG exists, and if it does exist, it is not clear that it applies to SLA. Additionally, research on the brain has found it very difficult to identify any areas or circuits

1

Speculation Direction

Psycholinguistic, Neurolinguistic, Cognitive Studies
Behavior ➤ Mechanism

Neurobiology of Learning
Mechanism ➤ Behavior

FIG. 1. Speculation direction.

that might constitute UG. On the other hand, neuroscience has produced considerable research that identifies the mechanisms for motivation and memory. These components have been shown to underlie a wide variety of learning tasks, and therefore, we chose to pursue the very conservative hypothesis that these mechanisms are ones that subtend second language learning.

Our approach is to describe the neurobiology for motivation, procedural knowledge, declarative knowledge, memory consolidation, and attention and then to speculate on how these neural mechanisms implement the acquisition and use of language. Our discussions range from the gross and cellular neuroanatomical to the behavioral levels. In the final chapter, we attempt to formulate a comprehensive neurobiology of SLA.

A word about the chapters. Psychological theory almost universally assumes that across individuals brain structure is homogeneous. Thus, most psychological research on learning proceeds on the notion that all brains are the same. The first chapter challenges this assumption because, from the perspective of neurobiology, brains are as different as faces. At the microlevel of neural structure and even at the gross level of sulci and gyri, each brain is unique. In the chapters on motivation, memory, and attention, we describe the neural systems as though they are uniform interindividually. However, it must be kept in mind that this uniformity is just a heuristic; the structure of each of the systems will vary across individuals. This variation has important implications for second language acquisition because it means that there are many ways to acquire language. In the second language teaching profession there has been a constant search for the "right way" to teach a language. A search for the right way entails the traditional psychological assumption of homogeneity. But because homogeneity does not exist in human brains, there can be no right way.

The second chapter describes how motivation can be reduced to the notion of "stimulus appraisal" and how it can be related to specific neural structures. Additionally, it shows how the concept of motivation is merely a higher order symbolic construction of what is achieved through the brain's reward system. All organisms have reward systems that tell them which stimuli to approach and which stimuli to avoid; this chapter attempts to show how motivation, as construed in second language research, can be understood as simply appraisal of the stimulus situation and the decision to approach or avoid. Additionally, the chapter indicates that motivation is not independent of cognition (as it is frequently treated in SLA research), but instead it is part of cognition, and therefore, there can be no "cognitive" approaches to SLA that do not include motivation.

Chapters 3, 4, and 5 deal with memory: procedural, declarative, and the processes of memory consolidation. A careful reading of these chapters and attention to the neurobiology will give the reader a detailed account of how these memory processes, which have been described in previous accounts of second language acquisition as metaphors, are implemented in the neural substrate. An important contribution that the neural perspective can provide is how these memory systems (declarative and procedural) are related and how information may be transmitted from one to another. This allows us to discuss, from a biological perspective, issues that have plagued the field such as the relationship between learning and acquisition, the phenomenon of fossilization, and the possibility of defossilization.

Chapter 6, on attention, has a dual task. The first is to come to grips with the notion of "attention" itself. At the level of psychology, attention has frequently been dealt with as a rather uniform phenomenon instantiated in a single mechanism, but from the perspective of the brain, attention appears to be distributed across many mechanisms. Joaquin Fuster (personal communication) suggested that the brain does not have an attention mechanism, but rather it has attention components in many mechanisms. The second task of this chapter is to describe the biology of those attention components. Therefore, this chapter is both a critique and a characterization of attention.

We have arranged the chapters in this book according to theme. We begin with an account of how all brains differ. This notion is essential in understanding variable success in second language learning. The second chapter is an account of motivation as the process which initiates and sustains learning. As just mentioned, chapters 3, 4, and 5 all concern memory, and 6 involves attentional processes that, like motivation, are important in modulating memory formation. Additionally, several themes from the SLA literature are treated in multiple chapters. For example, learning versus acquisition is discussed biologically in chapters 3 and 4; fossilization and defossilization are discussed in chapters 3 and 6, L2 rule learning is treated in chapters 3 and 4; L2 lexical acquisition is treated in chapters 4 and 5; and appraisal/motivation is discussed in chapters 1, 2, and 6.

TAXONOMY OF MEMORY

A major aspect of the neurobiology of learning involves memory, and three chapters of this book are devoted to memory processes. Therefore, it may be useful to provide taxonomy of memory here in the introduction in order to guide the neurobiology for discussions that are presented in chapters 3, 4, and 5. Figure 2 provides the standard hierarchical taxonomy of memory. Memory has been defined in both functional and temporal terms. With respect to the latter, memory has been broadly classified into working (short-term) and long-term memory (Fabbro, 1999; Fuster, 1995).

Working memory has traditionally been defined as memory that is held for short period of time (less than 20 seconds) in order to achieve success at a task. However, Fuster (personal communication) asserted that working memory has functions beyond its temporal duration. According to Fuster (1995), working memory can be defined by two criteria: a future perspective with emphasis on the execution of a future task, and its subservience to action such that it is memory for the sole pur-

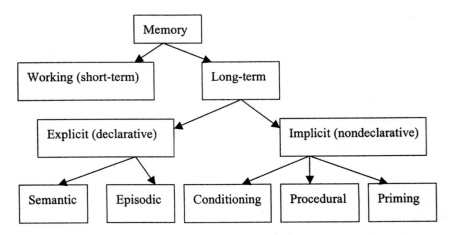

FIG. 2. Hierarchical classification of memory (based on Fabbro, 1999. Adapted with permission).

pose of accomplishing a task. Because the distinction between working memory and short-term memory is difficult to make, they are shown as one item in Figure 2. *Long-term memories* are those lasting for extended periods of time, from days, to weeks or for as long as months or years (Squire & Kandel, 2000).

Functionally, there are two major types of memory: declarative (or explicit) and nondeclarative (or implicit; see Fuster, 1995 for a review). These classifications sometimes assume different names such as memory with knowledge (i.e., declarative) and memory without knowledge (i.e., nondeclarative; Eichenbaum & Bodkin, 1999). Broadly defined, declarative memories are memories for facts and events, and nondeclarative memories are memories for habits, motor and perceptual skills, and emotional learning (Fuster, 1995; Squire & Kandel, 2000).

Declarative memory can be subclassified into semantic memory or memory for facts or encyclopedic knowledge of the world. These memories are not tied to any particular experience (Fabbro, 1999; Fuster, 1995; Squire & Kandel, 2000). The second category of declarative memory consists of episodic memories or recollections of past events or experiences, including the relevant temporal and spatial details of those events (Fuster, 1995). It is generally assumed that declarative memories can be recalled consciously (Aglioti, 1999; Fabbro, 1999; Milner, 1999; Tulving, 1972). All declarative memory is subtended by the hippocampal system and the neocortex.

Nondeclarative memory is subclassified into conditioning, procedural memory, and priming (Fabbro, 1999); or into skill and habit learning, emotional conditioning, and classical conditioning (Aglioti, 1999). Nondeclarative memories are subserved by both the hippocampal and the basal ganglia systems. Among these, procedural memory is largely supported by the basal ganglia (Graybiel, 1998; Hikosaka, Rand, Miyachi, & Miyashita, 1995; Joel & Weiner, 1998).

Declarative memory and nondeclarative memory have distinct characteristics. The classification depends on whether conscious introspection about the contents of the particular memory trace is present (Fabbro, 1999). Nondeclarative memory content cannot be accessed through conscious effort. Declarative memory, on the other hand, can be consciously recalled, represented, or verbalized (Aglioti, 1999; Fabbro, 1999). Nondeclarative memory, unlike declarative memory, is relatively inflexible and only available in contexts that are identical or very similar to the original learning situation (Aglioti, 1999). However, this also means that nondeclarative memory is more robust. It is spared and preserved in the elderly, whereas declarative memory deteriorates dramatically with aging (Aglioti, 1999). Finally, nondeclarative memory precedes declarative memory both phylogenetically and ontogenetically (Aglioti, 1999; Paradis, 1994).

Now let's take a brief look at the areas of the brain that are relevant to our discussion. Figure 3 is an attempt to capture all these areas in a single view. A brain cut down the middle is shown so that we can see the inside of the brain and part of the overlying right cerebral cortex. The areas that are particularly relevant to chapter 2, on motivation, are the amygdala, the nucleus accumbens, and the orbitofrontal cortex (OFC). Additionally, the neurotransmitter dopamine plays an important role in motivation. The cell bodies of origin for dopamine are in the midbrain and are indicated on the figure as the ventral tegmental area and the substantia nigra pars compacta. Procedural memory, as discussed in chapter 3, focuses on the caudate, the putamen, and the globus pallidus. Declarative memory, chapter 4, involves the hippocampus, and memory consolidation, chapter 5, is achieved through interaction between various areas in the neocortex and the hippocampus. As is seen in chapter 6, attention is distributed throughout the brain, but three regions can be identified as among those that are important to the substrate for this process: the dorsolateral prefrontal cortex, the parietal cortex, and the anterior cingulate. All these areas are rarely discussed in relation to language. Most people, if they are familiar with some aspect of language and the brain, have heard about Broca's area and Wernicke's area. These two regions certainly have something to do with language processing because Broca's area is part of the motor system and Wernicke's area is part of the auditory system. But when the task is to describe language learning, the central areas become those that subserve motivation, memory and attention; and therefore, it is these areas and their interconnections that are the central focus of this book.

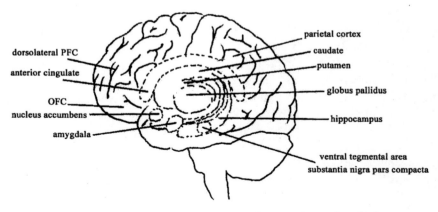

FIG. 3. Areas of the brain involved in learning (see text for explanation).

1   The Neurobiology of Aptitude

John H. Schumann

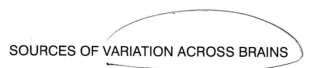

SOURCES OF VARIATION ACROSS BRAINS

The major thesis of this chapter is that all brains are different—as different as faces (Edelman, 1987, 1989, 1992) and that these differences have consequences for learning. The sources of variation among humans' brains are both genetic and epigenetic. I first examine the way genetic inheritance generates differences.

Each child receives roughly half the genes from its mother and half from its father. But the composition of the set of the parents' genes is different for each child, with the result that siblings are about 50% similar (Dunn & Plomin, 1990). Thus, we share about half our genes with our brothers and sisters. Of course, identical (monozygotic) twins are genetically the same, but fraternal twins (dyzygotic) share no more genetic material than ordinary siblings.

In terms of IQ, this genetic variation produces the following results. Identical twins' IQs correlate at about .86, fraternal twins have a correlation of about .60 and regular siblings have an IQ correlate of about .48. Environmental influences are estimated at .32 for regular siblings and .11 for monozygotic twins. Therefore, genetic influence on IQ for non-twins seems to be about .50 and environmental influence about .30 (Hamer & Copeland, 1998, Segal, 1999).

Edelman (1987, 1989, 1992) explained that genes do not specify the targets of all neurons (brain cells). Instead, they control the expression of adhesion molecules that cause cells to bind together and move along certain trajectories. These processes are largely stochastic and depend on the local mechanicochemical milieu in the embryo. A cell's ultimate location and connectivity is thus the result of the activity of the adhesion molecules and the chemical influences on the cell's history. This activity, called developmental selection, leads to brains that are similar in overall construction but which vary considerably at the level of

microstructure (i.e., circuitry formed among neurons, axons, and dendrites; Edelman, 1987, 1989, 1992).

A third source of variation is experiential selection (Edelman, 1987, 1989, 1992). Developmental selection establishes a "primary repertoire" (Edelman, 1987, 1989, 1992), which consists of neuronal groups whose connections, and thus basic circuitry, are formed by the activity of adhesion molecules during embryology. Postnatally, as the infant interacts with the environment, certain of these circuits match or resonate with the environmental input, and their synapses become strengthened. So in a very real sense, in the process of experiential selection, the environment selects the neuronal circuits in the brain that will subserve a particular signal or set of signals. Because each individual's environmental experience is different, experiential selection operating on the variation in the primary repertoire generates brains which, at the level of microanatomy, are even more different from one another. In addition to selection on the primary repertoire, growth in neural structure (i.e., growth of axons, dendrites, dendritic spines, and connections among them) is fostered by interaction between the environment and intrinsic growth mechanisms. This interaction generates additional variations across brains (Quartz & Sejnowski, 1997).

A fourth factor influencing variability in brains is a phenomenon called degeneracy (Edelman, 1987, 1989; Edelman & Tononi, 2000). Degeneracy comes about when there are two or more structurally different neural systems that can produce the same output. The structure of the alternate systems may differ from brain to brain.

Another source of variation involves the individual's development of preferences and aversions. This is actually a subform of experiential selection. The child is born with some innate biases. Homeostatic value is such a bias and serves to maintain stability in bodily systems (Edelman, 1989). It regulates hunger, thirst, warmth, heart rate, blood pressure, and so on. The individual will make efforts in the world to maintain a stasis in satiety, body temperature, and autonomic functions. Another innate bias system can be called sociostatic value, which relates to the tendency for all humans to seek out facial, vocal and tactile interaction with conspecifics. It is this bias that prepares human infants to acquire language by making the voices and faces of caregivers targets of automatic attention (Locke, 1995; Schumann, 1997).

Homeostatic and sociostatic value establish the basis for a form of experiential selection called somatic value (Edelman, 1987, 1992; Schumann, 1997), which consists of preferences and aversions, likes and dislikes that are not innate, but are acquired during the lifetime of the individual. This value system

or stimulus appraisal system (Leventhal & Scherer, 1987; Schumann, 1997) assesses internal and environmental stimuli on the basis of five criteria: novelty, pleasantness, goal significance, self and social image, and coping ability.

The novelty appraisal determines whether a stimulus or stimulus situation is new or whether it has been encountered before. Pleasantness appraisals assess whether the stimulus is pleasant in and of itself. The appraisals made on the goal dimension determine whether the stimulus situation will facilitate or hinder the individual in achieving his or her goals. The self and social image appraisals assess whether the stimulus situation is compatible with the individual's self-ideal and with the standards of other valued individuals. Coping involves one's ability to manage the situation (Scherer, 1984).

This appraisal system, which determines the emotional and motivational relevance of stimulus situations, is centered in the amygdala, the orbitofrontal cortex, and related structures (Rolls, 1999; Schumann, 1997). It influences the individual by incorporating into memory the individual's affective reactions to agents, events, and objects, and it then uses that information to evaluate future stimuli (Leventhal, 1984). The system emerges at birth and develops on the basis of experience in the world. Because each person's experience is different, the experience-dependent nature of the mechanism carves out highly variable neural preference systems across individuals (Schumann, 1997).

MANIFESTATION OF INDIVIDUAL DIFFERENCES

The previous section detailed the sources of interindividual variation in neural structure and physiology. In this section, individual differences in mental abilities are surveyed. The implicit hypothesis maintained here is that the variation in abilities manifest across individuals is caused by differences in the physical and chemical structure of the brain. Mental and physical abilities are demonstrated in behavior. We know that people differ because we see differences in their mental and physical production, and in their performance on tests. These differences must have a source, and I suggest that the source is the variation across brains. I am not able to empirically demonstrate this hypothesis; that awaits future developments in neuroimaging technology. But the current proposal will guide thinking about learning that takes into consideration neural and evolutionary principles; such considerations will allow us to prepare intelligently for empirical work.

Probably the most familiar manifestation of neurobiological differences is what emerges on peoples' performance on measures of intelligence. The standard IQ test indicates that general intelligence scores above 130 demonstrate su-

perior ability; a score of 100 marks average intelligence, and scores below 70 represent poor mental activity. Plomin (2001) pointed out that intelligence has come to mean many things, but there is something common to all tests of cognitive ability. The commonality is the g factor, and it is what is measured by the various cognitive subtests of the standard IQ batteries. Plomin argued that g may be the product of a link among more independent cognitive modules that was generated through evolution to subserve the challenges of domain general problem solving. The heritability of g is about 50% and therefore, differences in genes account for about half of g. The remainder may be the result of environmental experience or developmental selection.

Other tests that measure specialized abilities also demonstrate variation across individuals. An excellent example is the Modern Language Aptitude test (Carroll & Sapon, 1959). This instrument measures several abilities thought to underlie the capacity to acquire a second language. The components of this skill are the ability to rote memorize vocabulary quickly, the ability to distinguish and produce sounds, the ability to identify the grammatical function of a word in a sentence and then to locate a different word with a similar function in another sentence, and the ability to infer grammatical relations in an oral or written text. Individuals can score variably on the subtests, indicating that people differ in component abilities of second language learning aptitude.

Gardner (1993, 1999) developed a theory of multiple intelligences in which he is particularly interested in intelligence that is not part of g. He defined intelligences as "*a biopsychological potential to process information that can be activated in a cultural setting to solve problems or create products that are of value in a culture*" (1999, pp. 33–34). He argued that intelligences:

> are potentials—presumably neural ones—that will or will not be activated, depending upon the values of the particular culture, the opportunities available in that culture, and the personal decisions made by individuals and/or their families, school teachers, and others." (1999, pp. 33–34)

He focused on individual variation, arguing that "no two people have exactly the same kinds of minds, since we each assemble our intelligences in unique configurations" (p.150).

Gardner (1993, 1999) has identified seven intelligences: linguistic, logical-mathematical, musical, bodily-kinesthetic, spatial, interpersonal, and intrapersonal. Additionally, he is exploring the idea that there may be two others: naturalist intelligence and spiritual intelligence. Linguistic intelligence is the ability to acquire easily and effectively the use of sounds, words, and grammar orally and in the written form. It includes a sensitivity to codes and linguistic nuance at both the

sentence and text level. These abilities are employed to achieve one's goals in fields such as law, writing, and public speaking/oratory. Logical-mathematical intelligence involves the ability to learn and employ mathematical calculation and computation in solving problems, the ability to work logically through tasks, and a capacity to use traditional scientific procedure in defining, analyzing, and working through problems.

The next three intelligences are manifest especially in the arts. Musical intelligence is the ability to understand, appreciate, and compare and/or perform musical codes. Bodily-kinesthetic intelligence involves the ability to use parts of the body or the whole body in artistic and athletic performance, problem solving, material production, and technology. Spatial intelligence is the ability to conceptualize and orient to various special domains as manifest in talent for representing them (maps, painting), navigating them, abstracting and manipulating the patterns, orientations, and relationships. Interpersonal intelligence is the capacity to make accurate assessments of the intentions, and dispositions of others such that one can work successfully in relationships to achieve one's own and mutual goals. Intrapersonal intelligence is the ability understand one's own intentions, dispositions, motivations, strengths, and weaknesses and to use this information to effectively regulate one's intellectual, emotional, and social behavior.

Finally, Gardner investigates the possibility that humans may also have naturalistic intelligence and spiritual intelligence. Naturalistic intelligence involves special ability to recognize and classify things of the natural world (plants, animals, etc.) as well as other aspects of the environment (sounds, objects, measurements). Spiritual intelligence consists of an aptitude for examining and conceptualizing the nature of existence.

A particularly powerful manifestation of individual differences in brain structure comes from studies of Einstein's brain. Gardner (1993) provided a detailed study of Einstein's particular form of creativity, which he argued was the product of the scientist's remarkable logicomathematical and spatial intelligence.

Gardner pointed out that Einstein was object centered (rather than person centered like Freud). He was fascinated by objects and the relations among them. His father manufactured electrical appliances. Einstein found these machines fascinating and that interest extended to puzzles, wheels, and all things with moving parts. At 12, he was deeply impressed when he read a book on Euclidean geometry. At 16, he wondered whether a person moving alongside a light wave could exceed the speed of the wave. Later, he imagined a large box with a man inside it freefalling through space and wondered if the items in his pockets were taken out would they float freely in the box or would they fall to the bottom of the box.

Gardner went on to point out that Einstein had the ability to imagine configurations of objects in space, to mentally manipulate those configurations, and then to imagine the effect of the manipulations on the objects and their movement. Gardner says that Einstein was able to "integrate spacial imagery, mathematical formalisms, empirical phenomena, and basic philosophical issues" (p. 105).

Einstein's brain was preserved after his death and an examination of it showed that he had many more glial cells (support structures for neurons) than age-matched controls (Diamond, Scheibel, Murphy, & Harvey, 1985). Witelson, Kigar, and Harvey (1999) also studied his brain. They reasoned that the cognition Einstein required in the conceptualization of relativity involved "the generation and manipulation of three dimensional spatial images and the mathematical representation of concepts" (p. 2149). They also noted that the posterior parietal regions of the human brain seem to subserve "visuospatial cognition, mathematical ideation, and imagery of movement." (p. 2149). Therefore, they decided to study Einstein's parietal lobes to see whether they were different from those of control subjects.

They found that posterior limbs of his Sylvian fissure do not exist and the fissure joins the post-central sulcus. This architecture eliminates the parietal operculum which, in normal brains, lies between the postcentral sulcus and the posterior segment of the lateral sulcus. In addition, Einstein's parietal lobes were symmetrical, whereas those of most humans lack this symmetry. Each hemisphere in his brain was 15% larger than in the controls, and his parietal lobes were wider and more spherical than normal. The elimination of the parietal operculum expanded the area of the inferior parietal lobule in which visual, somatosensory, and auditory stimuli are integrated and where visuospatial and mathematical cognition as well as movement imagery are processed. The hypothesis that Witelson et al. entertain is that this hypertrophy had functional consequences allowing Einstein to cognize creatively in domains related to his scientific contributions.

One particularly salient manifestation of neurobiological variation is the abilities of savants and gifted children. Winner (2000) explained that savants typically have IQs between 40 and 70, but nevertheless have extraordinary ability in music, the visual arts or mathematics. Such savants, however, are rare. More typical savants have normal ability in one area but below normal aptitudes in all another intellectual or artistic domains. Winner also notes that prodigious savants, who are extremely rare, have one isolated but extremely high level of ability or skill.

Winner's (2000) focus is on gifted children. She described several cases. One is of a 3-year-old who learned to read by having his mother read two

books over and over to him as he pointed to the words. After he had done this about twelve times a day for 2 weeks, he had mastered English phoneme-grapheme relationships and then began to read extensively on his own. She also studied a child who, when he was 3 years old, knew whether or not any given number was a prime. Winner also described a 9-year-old boy who was fascinated with symbolic codes and learned to read musical scores and books on computer programming.

Winner pointed out that the gifted children tend to pursue their interest with passion. They spend vast amounts of time engaging environments related to their ability. They do not have to be encouraged by their parents; their motivation is intrinsic. Winner called this drive a "rage to master" (p. 40). This expression is similar to Plomin's (1999) characterization of the g factor as an appetite rather than an aptitude.

Winner cited research by Csikszentmihalyi, Rathunde, and Wholen (1993) where students who had exceptional talents in the visual arts or athletics were not necessarily academically talented. She argued that such results demonstrate the independence of IQ from, at least, these two areas of talent/ability.

A final source of evidence for variation across brains comes from research on the neural structure of monozygotic twins. Identical twins have the same genes, and therefore, if genes exclusively controlled brain structure, then we would expect that such twins' brains would be exactly the same. Research by Bartley, Jones, and Weinberger (1997) has shown that total brain size or volume is the same in monozygotic twins (but not dizygotic) and is therefore probably under genetic control. However, the gyral patterns of brains in monozygotic pairs are different, and this variable architecture must therefore be substantially influenced by epigenetic phenomena (i.e., developmental selection, experiential selection, and environmentally generated neural growth).

A DARWINIAN VIEW OF LEARNING

On the basis of interindividual differences in neuroanatomy and physiology and the variation in abilities across individuals, I argue for a selectionist view of learning. The basic notion is that the differences in brains are selected by the environment in the Darwinian sense. This leads to facilitated learning, and in many cases, to extraordinary expertise. From this view, for example, an individual may enter school with a particular neurohypertrophy for numerocity (caused by any of the phenomena as just described). The individual is then exposed to an environment in which mathematics and mathematical reasoning are available. This environment selects the neuronal groups, assemblies, en-

sembles, and maps that constitute the individual's hypertrophy. These brain systems respond to the environment (exposure to and instruction in mathematics), and the acquisition of mathematical knowledge is facilitated. A person without such a neural hypertrophy has to make much greater effort to learn and requires more time (and perhaps instruction) to acquire similar mathematical knowledge. The person with the brain systems supporting extraordinary mathematical ability might someday achieve high expertise in this field, which may be exercised in a career in mathematics, engineering, physics, or computing.

Probably the most obvious example of selection on differences in neuronal systems can be seen in athletic ability. Motor coordination governed by cortical, basal ganglia, and cerebellar mechanisms differ across individuals. Some people may have a general hypertrophy for motoric acuity; others may have more specific strengths that can be selected by a particular athletic enterprise. What becomes clear is that the neural strengths must exist in an environment where they are useful, valued, or needed in order for them to be selected. For example, in a society that does not permit women to engage in athletic activities, those young women with a neural hypertrophy that would subserve a high level of athletic ability would not be selected by the environment for this talent.

A selectionist view of learning makes evolutionary sense. The evolution of nervous systems, which vary substantially across individuals, permits environmental selection on that variation. Environments frequently change rapidly. With a diverse set of nervous systems available, some subset of individuals is likely to have the appropriate neurobiology to respond to the change. (The ability to respond allows those individuals to thrive in their lifetimes, making them objects for sexual selection and thus the spread of their genes [Miller, G., 2000]). Under extraordinary conditions, which may be life threatening to a species, having substantial diversity across nervous systems increases the chance for the survival of some individuals.

Evidently, there is an ant colony that extends from the Mexican border in California to San Luis Obispo. Here ants with their various specializations—workers, warriors, and so on—provide expertise to support this vast empire. We might also conceive of the human species as a vast colony. It began with some migration out of Africa and then some major cultural development in the Fertile Crescent. From there, over the past several thousand years, the colony has spread throughout the whole world.

What has made this expansion possible? I would suggest that the main contribution is the genetic and epigenetic diversity in the human population. Through mutation, sexual recombination, developmental selection, degeneracy, and experiential selection, our species produces individuals that vary

enormously from each other. The second contribution has been the human ability to make symbolic reference (Deacon, 1997). This ability allowed the development of culture in which adaptation to the environment could take place without genetic assimilation. Culture allowed the development of tools for adaptation (clothes, housing, agriculture, weapons, etc.). The diversity in our species produces brains that are as different as faces. Therefore, when we encountered an environmental challenge, there were usually one or more individuals who could invent a cultural/technological response to it and then provide that response to other individuals who lacked that creativity. Because humans were a symbolic species with language at their disposal, they were also able to teach and learn cultural innovations that allowed them to adapt and survive in the changing environment. In this way, our species has spread across the planet.

Thus, it may be that variation in brains is what has permitted humans to survive in almost every possible econiche. As previously mentioned, with the development of culture, the environment changes much more rapidly. Those who can respond will thrive. For example, individuals who were once considered socially awkward have frequently been able to thrive in the new computer culture. Their computational expertise may constitute a sexual ornament and fitness indicator resulting in these genes being spread (Miller, G., 2000). We may discover someday a cultural niche in which the cognitive and social characteristics of autistic people will be selected (perhaps for some aspects of space travel) and these individuals will thrive. Variation in neural structure is sometimes an asset in a particular environment, sometimes it is neutral, and sometimes it is a deficit. Variation can lead to success or pathology, or it may have no effect at all.

The notion of selection as a cause of learning and expertise is counterintuitive. We see ourselves as intentional beings with plans, goals, and desires. We see ourselves as choosing to learn, choosing a field to master. Thus, the notion of selection is contrary to our experience. The inherent lack of control often makes it difficult to understand evolution, where variation in individuals allows some to survive and flourish and other to die off—and this happens without a goal, intelligent design, or agency. Therefore, we are likely to be suspicious of an idea that claims that we know what we know because the sources of that knowledge have selected us.

Perhaps selection is most obvious in cases of mastery of some form of knowledge or skill by very young children, as in the cases presented earlier by Winner (2000). It is unlikely that a 3-year-old initially had the goal to discover whether any number was a prime or not. A recent story in the *The New*

York Times (Steinglass, 2001) told of a boy in Togo, West Africa, who became a pianist and participates in international competitions. When he was 3 years old, his parents (both doctors) bought a piano for his sister. It was soon clear that he had extraordinary musical talent. By the time he was 9, he could play Beethoven's First Piano Concerto, at 12 he won a scholarship to a music festival in the United States and a year later he was a finalist in that festival's piano competition. The author of the article points out that in all of Togo there may be only 10 pianos. The young man was fortunate to have access to one of them and to have had access to a dedicated and talented piano teacher. However, we can imagine that among his age cohort in Togo there may have been one or more Togans that had the brains and musculoskeletal systems that would have allowed them to become concert pianists, but in their environments, there was no piano or piano teacher to select them. Thus, their neural hypertrophy would go unnoticed and undeveloped.

But our nervous systems, as well as being objects of selection by the environment, are also capable of intentional, goal-oriented activity. This is the activity of which we are conscious. Scarr and McCarthy (1983), in examining individual differences among children, describe genotype→experience effects. They present a theory in which an individual's genes interact with the environment. The first interaction involves passive effects, in which the parents, whose genes the child inherits, provide the major environmental input to the child. In the second kind of interaction, the individual chooses and/or creates environments that are compatible with his or her talents. The third way genotype interacts with the environment is through the evocation of responses from the environment. Evocative effects are those that an individual elicits from others. Scarr and McCarthy (1983) noted that smiley, happy infants evoke more positive responses from family and caretakers than do passive or cranky infants. They also point out how people with mechanical ability receive responses from technological environments that are very different from the responses experienced by those who lack mechanical ability. Another powerful example (Scarr, 1996) is how people who are physically attractive evoke different responses from other individuals in their environment than do unattractive people. Lemley (2000) wrote that:

> Landmark studies show that attractive males and females not only garner more attention from the opposite sex, they also get more affection from their mothers, more money at work, more votes from the electorate, more leniency from judges, and are generally regarded as more kind, competent, healthy, confident, and intelligent than their big-nosed, weak-chinned counterparts. (p. 44)

The argument I am making is that brains vary just as faces do, and the environment selects on brains just as it does on faces.

What Scarr described as evocation of environmental response is quite similar to my notion of selection. Scarr and McCarthy (1983) argued that "individuals select and evoke experiences that are directly influenced by their genotypes" (p. 430). I alter and elaborate their position in the following way: Individuals select [=choose] and evoke [=are selected by] experiences [=environments] that are directly influenced by [=resonate with] their genotypes [and the neural products of developmental selection, experiential selection, and somatic selection].

Selection has another dimension. An individual with a hypertrophy for particular knowledge or skill (basketball, chess, history, chemistry) will develop procedural and/or declarative knowledge consisting of responses that manifest automatically under certain conditions. Collections of such automatized knowledge systems, once developed, then stand as a set of variations on which the environment can select. The idea of expertise or skill is to be able to respond automatically (i.e., without overt intention) to environmental conditions that present themselves. So individuals appear to intentionally develop repertoires of automatic knowledge and skill in order to manifest expertise when environmental conditions (sports, games, information provision) call it forth (i.e., select it). Thus, we see environmental selection on unique strengths of nervous systems, which are acquired through genetic or epigenetic processes, and selection on nervous systems as individuals have intentionally developed them through learning.

This position is very much in the tradition of Gardner's (1993, 1999) theory of multiple intelligences, but whereas Gardner (and others such as Sternberg, 1985) is concerned with the nature of intelligence, this view is concerned with the nature of learning. The two perspectives are obviously related. Gardner identified eight forms of intelligence: linguistic, logical-mathematical, bodily kinesthetic, musical, spatial, interpersonal, intrapersonal, and naturalist. He sees these as constituting largely independent mental modules. The view expressed here is somewhat different. I believe that the processes of cell division, developmental selection, experiential selection, neural construction, degeneracy and stimulus appraisal conspire to produce the several intelligences that Gardner proposes. However, these processes also generate hypertrophies and hypotrophies within the various intelligences that promote and inhibit the acquisition of knowledge and skill within the neuronal circuits that subserve the various forms of intelligence.

These neural variations may provide individuals with small and subtle or large and profound advantages and deficits. Additionally, the position presented here is based more explicitly on neural and evolutionary considerations. Nevertheless, there is nothing contradictory between this view and Gardner's. They both represent contemporary efforts to understand learning and intelligence from the perspective of individual differences. In both views, interindividual variations are not seen as exceptions or noise, as in traditional psychology (Miller, G., 2000), but rather they are considered as a universal basis on which theories of human cognition must be built.

Gardner (1999) pointed out that the notion of a singular intelligence as measured by IQ tests was "formulated largely in terms of the capacities needed to exist in a certain kind of European or American school one century ago" (pp. 213–214). Schools require a kind of academic (largely linguistic and logico-mathematical) intelligence, and school environments select for it. The question then becomes how does society select for other intelligences? What institutions, programs, and environments select and nurture musical, spatial, body-kinesthetic, intrapersonal, interpersonal, and naturalist intelligences. Of course, some aspects of these intelligences are also features of the academic domain. But where societies value other intelligences, they provide environments for their selection and development. An appropriate question to ask is what are these environments. Just because we are using the word *intelligence*, we should not assume it is the domain of the schools. Schools are environments that require predominantly linguistic and mathematical intelligence. It is important to recognize where and how society develops and exploits other intelligences. It would appear that the cultural responses to neurally based variation in human abilities have been distributed across institutions. Therefore, various organizations, institutions, and practices (scouts, church-related activities, 4-H programs, the YMCA, sports teams, local departments of recreation, etc.) participate in the identification, nurture, and use of the range of abilities which result from variation in brains.

Differences in Brains and Differences in Aptitude for Second Language Acquisition

The issue of aptitude has special relevance for second language acquisition. As mentioned earlier, studies of aptitude among second language learners indicate that such an ability does indeed exist and that it has several sub-

components. The first component is the ability to perceive, code and produce the sounds of the second language. The second is the ability to rapidly and accurately acquire the meanings of the target language words. Generally, this is manifest in the ability to associate the words in the target language with translation equivalents in one's native language. The third component involves sensitivity to the grammatical function of words in a sentence. It is found in the ability to identify the grammatical function of a word in one sentence and then to identify a different word in another sentence that has the same function. The final component consists of the ability to identify grammatical patterns and their meanings in an oral or written text.

Conceivably individuals may vary in their ability on any of these subcomponents. A particular neural architecture might support the associative learning of target words and their native equivalents but may have no effect on one's ability to perceive grammatical patterns in the input. Similarly, an individual might have particularly good ability to imitate target language sounds, but may not necessarily have particular talent in lexical acquisition. Additionally, some individuals may be able to express their ability for lexical learning and grammatical learning from written texts more efficiently and effectively than from oral input. The opposite might also be true—some learners may have abilities that make them more comfortable practicing the language orally rather than visually.

Given these differences across individuals, it would be difficult to argue that there is any "right" way to teach a foreign language. Individuals generally need to learn to speak and comprehend, to read and to write. They will have to be able to perceive sounds and produce them, to learn words and how to order them and inflect them. A single individual might have neural substrate that supports all of these activities, some of the activities, or none of these activities. For there to be a "correct" way to teach a foreign language, would mean that all brains are the same with respect to that method. However, as previously discussed, brains vary, and therefore, people learn differently. This has important implications for a language teaching methodology. It means that one will never find a method for teaching a second language that will make the process rapid and the results uniform across learners. Good teachers provide general guidelines and direction; they remain informed about developments in their fields; they introduce innovations where appropriate, and evaluate their results. Second language learning is an 8 to 12 year enterprise, and ultimate proficiency will vary across individuals depending on variation in their aptitudes and variation in their motivation/stimulus appraisal.

A Note on Teaching

The evolutionary and neurobiological considerations presented in this chapter suggest a perspective on teaching. Because the task of all education and much medical practice is to make changes in an individual's nervous system, teaching may be viewed as a form of medical intervention.

In medical practice, treatments or medications affect people differently. The reason for this is that bodies of individuals differ in their anatomy and physiology. Some treatments find responders who benefit from the intervention; some patients react negatively to the treatment, and with others, the intervention has no effect at all. Because all brains are different, teaching works in the same way. Therefore, there can be no correct way to teach anything.

From the perspective of evolutionary selection, schools can be seen as playing a special role. Educational institutions require students to take a range of subjects. This is done for several reasons. The first is to provide important basic and specialized knowledge and skill in literary and numeracy. The second is to provide a broad exposure to other information so that the students will be able to thrive in the work world. The third is to produce well-educated people. The fourth and the fifth reasons relate to implicit functions of which education institutions themselves may be largely unaware.

A broad educational curriculum provides a varied environment, which increases the opportunity that an individual's particular neural variation might be selected. In other words, a wide range of curricular offerings (and requirements) increases the chances that a student will come in contact with an area of knowledge or skill that resonates with his or her unique neural structure. Such a resonance and selection allows an individual to develop expertise, which can then be used as a sexual ornament/fitness indicator both to attract a mate and to allow thrival in somatic time. The mental acuity, which is selected by the educational environment, may be passed on to offspring if it is genetically based. However, if the hypertrophy is the result of epigenetic factors (such as developmental or experiental selection) it would not be inherited. Of the three processes that characterize evolution by natural selection (variation, selection, inheritance), only the first two are operate in the processes which are epigenetic.

CONCLUSION

Evolution has no design; it produces biological structures guided by no goal or plan. Humans, however, can and do design; they do act according to plans to achieve particular goals. The environment selects on variation in brains, and intentional brains choose environments with which to engage to achieve a goal according to a plan. Thus, environments attract brains to them, and brains deliberately seek out resonant environments with which to interact. Therefore, humans operate in the world by selection and by intention. We are passively selected and actively choose. We are conscious of choosing, but are generally not conscious of the fact that environments are selecting us (i.e., our mental and physical abilities).

Based on neurobiological and evolutionary considerations, this chapter has focused on learning as a process of selection on the variation in human neuroanatomy and physiology. This position does not deny that learning is also the product of individual intention and choice, but one is likely to choose a field of expertise because an appetite for it is engendered by an aptitude that is selected by the environment.

2   The Neurobiology of Motivation

John H. Schumann
Lee A. Wood

SUSTAINED DEEP LEARNING

This chapter offers a neurobiological perspective on motivation as the basis for sustained deep learning (SDL) (Schumann, 1997). This type of learning is called sustained because it takes an extended period of time to achieve—often several years. And it is called deep because when the process is completed, the learner is considered proficient or an expert. This kind of learning must be distinguished from what is known as canalized learning. Canalized processes are those that have been selected in evolution and for which an individual is innately equipped. Examples are learning to see, to walk, and to attend to faces and voices. Such learning is inevitable in all normal individuals and seems to occur with a minimum of environmental input. SDL must also be distinguished from the type of learning that is studied in most psychological research. In psychological experiments, participants typically learn material unrelated to their goals and are tested on it after relatively short periods of time.

The kind of learning we are talking about requires the brain to become a specialist in something for which it has no specialization. Therefore, such learning involves a great deal of individual variation. In a particular area, some individuals may become highly proficient, others may acquire less proficiency, and still others may acquire no knowledge or skill in the area at all. Examples of such learning are things such as becoming a neuroscientist, a chef, a tennis player, an accountant, a violinist, and architect, or a speaker of a second language. In the perspective we will present, second language acquisition will be analyzed as a paradigm case of sustained deep learning.[1]

THE THEORY

Value

The theory of learning presented here is rooted in the biological notion of value (Edelman, 1992; Schumann, 1997). Value is a bias that leads an organism to certain preferences and enables it to choose among alternatives (Damasio, 1994). Some aspects of value are so important that evolution has selected for them and they have become innate. Value is the basis for all activity; we perceive, move, cognize, and feel on the basis of value. We can distinguish between three types of value: homeostatic, sociostatic, and somatic.

Homeostatic Value

Homeostatic value (Edelman, 1992) involves preferences that promote an organism's survival and thrival in the world. It is a biological tendency for an organism to maintain its physiological system within a certain range, to move outside that range to survive, and to return to that range to thrive. Homeostatic systems control such things as respiration, heart rate, body temperature, satiation, eliminatory functions, and sexual drive.

Sociostatic Value

Sociostatic value (Schumann, 1997) might be seen as an interactional instinct. It involves inborn tendencies to interact with conspecifics, to pay attention to faces, voices, and body position, to make hypotheses about the intentions and dispositions of others, and to seek attachment and social affiliation.

Somatic Value

Somatic value (Edelman, 1992; Friston, Tononi, Reek, Sporns, & Edelman, 1994; Schumann, 1997) involves preferences and aversions acquired in the lifetime of the individual through experience, socialization, enculturation, and educa-

---

[1]In this model, second language acquisition is seen as nothing special. Just as any other form of sustained deep learning, it results from appraisal-generated mental and motor activity. However, the model says nothing about how a second language is organized in the brain. A second language may have a neural organization that is different from that of other subjects such as mathematics or history.

tion. It is biased by innate homeostatic and sociostatic value, and appears to be particularly sensitive to early experience because of heightened neural plasticity early in life, but it is subject to modification throughout life due to continued but attenuated plasticity.

Memory for Value

As an organism moves through the world, it encounters various stimulus situations. It experiences the emotional impact of these stimuli in terms of their relevance to its homeostatic, sociostatic, and somatic value systems. It incorporates into its memory (schematic emotional memory [Leventhal, 1984] or value category memory [Edelman, 1992]) the characteristics of the stimulus situation and their relevance to its goals, its ability to adapt, its hedonic sense, and in higher organisms, its sense of self. This memory then becomes part of the value system used in evaluation of subsequent stimuli.

Determining Value

Psychologists have studied the kinds of appraisals or assessments individuals make of stimulus events to determine value. Several models have been proposed and there is considerable congruence among them. Scherer's (1984) taxonomy seems to provide a list of dimensions that are sufficiently broad to capture those characteristics of stimuli that constitute emotional significance for an individual and at the same time to capture the range of dimensions suggested by other researchers. He suggested that the emotional relevance of stimuli is assessed on the basis of novelty, pleasantness, and relevance to the individual's goals or needs, ability to cope, and compatibility with the individual's self and social image.

The novelty assessment determines whether the stimulus has been experienced before or whether it is new. The pleasantness dimension determines whether the stimulus situation is intrinsically pleasant or enjoyable for its own sake. The goal/need appraisal assesses whether or not the stimulus event is relevant to the individual's goals or needs and whether it is likely to promote or interfere with their achievement. Coping potential appraisals assess how the stimulus will affect the individual's ability to manage the demands of the situation. Coping potential assessments are essentially assessments of the individual's aptitude vis-a-vis the stimulus situation. Self and social compatibility appraisals determine whether engagement with the stimulus event will be enhancing of one's self image in terms of one's ideal self or enhancing of one's social image in terms of the expectations of valued others (Leventhal & Scherer, 1987; Scherer, 1984).

The Function of Stimulus Appraisals.   The stimulus appraisals compute the emotional relevance and motivational significance of stimulus events in relation to information stored in value category memory based on past experience. The appraisals generate emotions such as joy, happiness, fear, anger, and shame (Gehm & Scherer, 1988), and these emotions lead to action tendencies (Frijda, 1987; Frijda, Knipers, & ter Schure, 1989), such as, the readiness to undertake mental or motor behaviors in relation to stimulus.

THE MECHANISM

The neural mechanism proposed to subserve stimulus appraisal consists of the amygdaloid nuclei in the anterior temporal lobes on the sides of the brain (hereafter, amygdala), the orbitofrontal cortex (above the orbits of the eyes), and the body proper (the autonomic nervous system, the endocrine system, and the musculoskeletal system; see Fig. 2.1). Actual appraisals seem to be made in circuits in and related to the amygdala and the orbitofrontal cortex, but these two structures are connected to the peripheral nervous system where the appraisal causes a bodily state (called a somatic marker by Damasio, 1994). This bodily state is an emotion that is communicated to the brain as a feeling (Damasio, 1994). On the basis of the feeling, personal and social decisions are made. When there have been frequent associations between appraisals and bodily states, the resultant somatic markers can become centrally represented in the brain itself, obviating the need for processing in the peripheral nervous system (Brothers, 1995; Damasio, 1994).

Evidence that this neural system subserves stimulus appraisal comes from three sources:

1. observations of deficits in stimulus appraisal that occur when the amygdala or the orbitofrontal cortex are damaged in either animals or humans
2. responses from neurons in animal brains that have electrodes implanted in these structures
3. activation in these areas observed in neural imaging research (e.g., PET, fMRI).

Neurobiological research has shown that the amygdala, which is located in the temporal lobes on the sides of brain, is important in assessing positive or

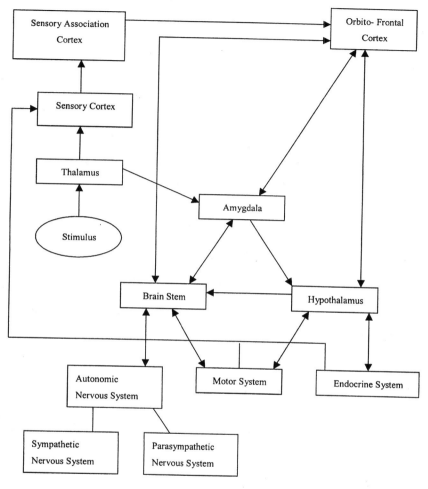

FIG. 2.1. The neural system for stimulus appraisal (from Schumann, 1997).

negative value of stimuli. Humans with bilateral amygdala damage fail to respond to normal fearful stimuli: threatening faces, instruments and agents, loss
of money (in simulated gambling tasks), and unusual objects in their environment. They are also unable to make normal character judgments in the basis of
facial expression, and they have a tendency to judge objects (e.g., paintings)

positively that normals evaluate negatively (Adophs & Tranel, 1999; Adolphs, Tranel, & Damasio, 1998; Adolphs, Tranel, Damasio, & Damasio, 1994; Baxter & Murray, 2002; LeDoux, 1996). Research also indicates that the amygdala plays a role in enhancing the consolidation of memories and therefore, it is important in learning (Hamann, Ely, Grafton, & Kilts, 1999; Ferry, Roozendaal, & McGaugh, 1999; McGaugh, Roozendaal, & Cahill, 2000; Paré, Collins, & Pelletier, 2002).

The orbitofrontal cortex is located in the front of the brain above the orbits of the eyes. It seems to be involved in appraisals related to somatic value. This part of the brain was a late development phylogenetically; it is also slow in ontogentic development, and it is not fully functional until the second decade of life. This appraisal area is important in the preferences and aversions that are acquired from socialization and education. Patients with damage to the orbitofrontal cortex have their deficits in personal and social decision-making and in producing appropriate social behavior. They have difficulty maintaining and achieving goals. These patients have severe difficulty in deciding among alternatives because they get no feedback or gut feeling from their peripheral nervous system to help them restrict decision-making to a limited set of alternatives. They seem to lose the behavioral control engendered by socialization, education, and enculturation. They frequently behave inappropriately in social situations, using foul language, associating with unsavory characters, and generally disregarding social mores. These patients have been reported to have exaggerated and inaccurate senses of their own abilities and qualities. Behavior that intact individuals consider risky or actually dangerous and to be avoided does not affect orbitofrontal patients in the same way, and thus the patients are more willing to engage in such behavior (Anderson, Bechara, Damasio, Tranel, & Damasio, 1999; Bechara, Damasio, & Damasio, 2000; Damasio, 1994; Schumann, 1997, 2001b).

The body proper or the peripheral nervous system is the third component in the neurobiological stimulus appraisal mechanism. Here, projections from the amygdala and the orbitofrontal cortex that interact with the autonomic nervous system, the endocrine system, and the muscuoloskeletal system foster positive or negative body states (once again, a gut feeling) that guide appropriate behavior. Thus, we literally think with our bodies—the body proper is a component in our cognition (Damasio, 1994). See Fig. 2.1.

MENTAL AND MOTOR FORAGING

To elaborate this neurobiolgical model of SDL, we consider three additional notions that support a brain-based view of learning. First, emotion and cognition are not separated neurobiology to the degree they are in psychology and cognitive science. The cognition involved in effective learning and behavior would be impossible without emotion, affect, or motivation to initiate and sustain it. Second, many cognitive systems may be evolutionary adaptations of motor systems. In neurobiology there is the notion of "up from movement" (Calvin, 1996, p. 152) where cognitive processes are seen as higher order functions of motor processes. These processes may operate on motor circuits or on neural networks that run parallel to those circuits. The third principle, is related to the second. Here learning can be seen as a form of mental foraging, which may engage the same neural systems that organisms use when foraging to feed or to mate (Schumann, 2001a).

When an animal sets out to feed or mate, it is because there has been a change in its homeostatic value system. Hunger is signaled by mechanisms in the hypothalamus that respond to low glucose levels. With regard to mating, a female goes into estrous and male becomes responsive via olfactory perception of pheromones, visual perception of the female, or auditory perception of mating calls. The changes in the animal's homeostasis cause it to undertake motor activity to achieve a goal—feeding or mating. When a human learner generates the desire to acquire some knowledge or skill, that desire also constitutes a goal that will require motor and mental activity to achieve.

This brings us to the latest part of our work on the possible neural substrate for learning. It goes beyond the model previously proposed and is more speculative. It recognizes that learning involves movement or motor activity and that it is goal directed. So we suggest that learning may be a form of mental or intellectual foraging involving motor activity to acquire knowledge or skill. Based on the neurobiological literature on the circuitry mediating the translation of motivational stimuli into adaptive motor responses (Kalivas, Churchill, & Klitenick, 1993) and the neurobiological literature on information processing in the brain's motor systems (Houk, Davis, & Beiser, 1995), we hypothesize a neural system for mental foraging. The goal for learning is generated in the limbic and paralimbic circuits involving the orbitofrontal cortex and the amygdala and is based on the individual's positive appraisal of the skill or knowledge to be acquired. The amygdala and orbitofrontal areas project to a motor area of the brain called the basal ganglia, which has both a ventral and dorsal aspect. The appraisal regions of the brain project to ventral basal ganglia, specifically the shell of the nucleus accumbens (NAs), which is innervated by dopamine (DA) from the ventral tegmental area (VTA) in the midbrain. The NAs then connects to the ventromedial ventral pallidum (VPm) (Deutch, Bourdelais, & Zahm,

1993; Heimer, Alheid, & Zahm, 1993; Mogenson, Brudzynski, Wu, Yang, & Yim, 1993). See Fig. 2.2.

The circuit in Fig. 2.2, holds the incentive motive or goal over time (Kalivas, Churchill, & Klitenick, 1993), probably in the form emotional memory (Leventhal, 1984) or value category memory (Edelman, 1992). Additionally, appraisal information from the amygdala and orbitofrontal cortex will modulate the intensity of the incentive motive, either increasing or decreasing it in relation to the assessment of the current stimulus situation.

From the VPm the circuit projects to the mediodorsal thalamus (MD) and from there to the prelimbic area of the prefrontal cortex (area 32) and then to the motor segment of the nucleus accumbens, the core (NAc), and the dorsolateral ventral pallidum (VP1). The VP1 projects to a midbrain locomotor region called the pedunculopontine nucleus (PPN), which then projects to brainstem motor nuclei that connect to the spinal cord (Deutch et al., 1993;

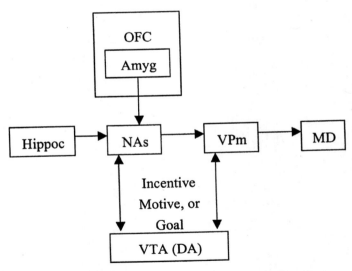

FIG. 2.2. The mechanism for generating the incentive motive or goal.
OFC = Orbitofrontal Cortex
Amyg = Amygdala
Hippoc = Hippocampus
NAs = Nucleus accumbens, shell
VPm = Ventromedial ventral pallidum
MD = Mediodorsal thalamus
VTA = Ventral tegmental area
DA = Dopamine

Heimer et al., 1993; Kalivas et al., 1993; Mogenson et al., 1993; Skinner & Garcia-Rill, 1993). This circuit, illustrated in Fig. 2.3, allows motivation to generate motor activity to achieve the organism's goal. It is probably also the circuit involved in the generation of foraging behaviors (Montague, Dayan, Pearson, & Sejnowski, 1995; Robbins & Everitt, 1996).

It is through this system the learner engages in motor and mental foraging. He or she motorically moves through the environment to do things to acquire the language. The learner may go to class, study vocabulary, do grammar exercises, listen to tapes, talk to native speakers, memorize dialogues or any number of things that she believes will facilitate learning the language. Essentially this system subserves the behaviors that have been described in the learning strategies literature (O'Malley & Chamot, 1990; Oxford, 1990). The learner's appraisal system evaluates these stimulus situations according to whether they are novel or pleasant, whether they are enhancing one's goal and one's self and social image, and whether they are within one's ability to cope (Scherer, 1984). The mechanism that makes these appraisals consists, once again, of the amygdala, the orbitofrontal cortex (see Fig. 2.1), and also includes the peripheral nervous system (the autonomic, endocrine and musculoskeletal systems; Damasio, 1994; Schumann, 1997). If the learner perceives that the stimulus situation is predictive of reward, that is, if he or she appraises the learning situation positively on one or more of the men-

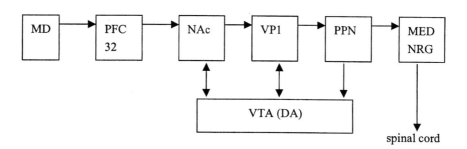

FIG. 2.3. The mechanism for generating mental and motor activity for learning.
PFC = Prefrontal cortex, area 32
NAc = Nucleus accumbens, core
VP1 = Dorsolateral ventral pallidum
PPN = Pedunculopontine nucleus
MED & NRG = Brainstem motor nuclei (medioventral medullary locomotor region, nucleus reticularis gigantocellularis)

tioned dimensions such that he or she feels his or her goal to learn the language has been served, then circuits in the dorsal basal ganglia come into play. Dopamine (DA) is released from the VTA and the substantia nigra (SN) into the striatum enabling the learner-forager to learn and remember the situations that were predictive of reward in the sense that they facilitated acquiring something of the language. This part of the learning mechanism is illustrated in Fig. 2.4 (Graybiel, Aosaki, Flaherty, & Kimura, 1994; Houk, Adams, & Barto, 1995; Schultz, 1997; Schultz, Dayan, & Montague, 1997; Schultz, Romo, Ljungberg, Mirenowicz, Hollerman, & Dickinson, 1995).

DA neurons in the VTA and the SNc, which receive highly convergent input from many areas of the brain, encode information about reward and communicate that information to areas such as the striatum, the NA, and the frontal cortex, which are involved in motivation and goal directed behavior (Schultz, 1997). The DA neurons constitute feature detectors that determine whether the stimulus situation is predictive of reward in terms of achieving the organism's goals. A positive signal is recorded if the stimulus situation provides an unpredicted re-

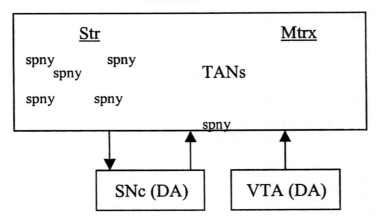

striatum

FIG. 2.4. The mechanism for remembering situations or actions that facilitate or predict learning.
Str = striosomes
spny = medium spiny neurons
TANs = tonically activated neurons
Mtrs = matrix
SNc = substantia nigra, pars compacta

ward or if the reward is greater than expected. In both these situations, the organism (in our case, a learner) learns that the stimulus is facilitative of its goal. If the organism makes a prediction that the event will be aversive, and it turns out to be rewarding, learning will take place. In all these situations, DA activity is enhanced. Finally, when an organism predicts reward and it fails to occur, DA activity is depressed (Schultz, 1997).[2]

One can see how this mechanism would be important in both foraging for food and foraging for knowledge. In both cases, the forager must be able to learn and later recall those stimulus situations that lead to the goal or—to put it another way—that fulfill the incentive motive. To have to start each foraging expedition from scratch would be defeating. What a successful forager/learner may be doing is taking actions that result in increased DA activity and avoiding those that result in decreased DA activity (Schultz, 1997). On the other hand, what the learner may be doing is learning and remembering actions that result in increased DA activity in order to repeat those actions to increase learning. The forager/learner may also remember those situations/actions in which there was depressed DA, and avoid those situations in the future.

Primary reinforcers such as food consumption, sex, or the acquisition of knowledge or skill may be preceded by a series of stimuli or stimulus situations that predict the eventual primary reinforcer. Spiny neurons in the striasomes of the striatum receive motivational information that is communicated via DA inputs and TANS to output neurons in the matrix (Fig. 2.4; Graybiel et al., 1994; Houk et al., 1995; Schultz et al., 1995; see chap. 3 for more detailed description of this system). The striatal spiny neurons detect contexts that are predictors of reward. DA neurons project back to the same striatal neurons that send them input, and this loop allows the identification of antecedent stimuli that predict the same reward. Thus, this system can identify chains of reinforcers, ultimately leading to reward (Houk et al, 1995). A good example of such chains might be links in an internet system. An example from language learning might be a teaching assistant who directs a learner to a language laboratory that has a materials guide that lists a CD-ROM that provides a series of exercises that facilitate, for the learner, the acquisition of the perfective/imperfective distinction in Russian.

The series of reinforcers raises the credit assignment problem (Houk et al., 1995). How does the organism ultimately determine and remember which of

[2]Rolls (1999) suggested that the release of dopamine into the striatum may be more related to the initiation of action than to the expectation of reward. He argued that evidence for this issue would come from experiments that would demonstrate that dopamine release also occurs in response to aversive stimuli to initiate avoidance behaviors.

the earlier contexts actually were predictive of reward? This might be especially difficult in long sequences over long periods of time. We know that we often believe a particular context is predictive of reward, but later we may see that, in fact, the stimulus event did not lead to the primary reinforcer that was expected. For example, one may read an article that one feels will help him or her get the knowledge he or she wants. One finds a reference in that article which one thinks will bring him or her even closer to that knowledge. One gets the second article, reads it and finds it was too technical to understand and thus did not provide the desired knowledge. Here one would receive the DA response for the prediction of reward, but the context (i.e., the article), is not, after all, rewarding. How the brain goes back and reassigns credit has not yet been settled in the neurobiological research (but see Houk et al., 1995) and remains an important question for future research.

Finally, we assume the positive appraisal of the language learning situation results in conscious or unconscious attention to the components of the language involved: sounds, words, inflections, order of elements, pragmatic features. The positive hedonic state generated in the limbic circuits (amygdala, etc.) causes acetylcholine (ACh) to be released from the nucleus basalis of Meynert (NBM) (Weinberger, 1995). The ACh is distributed in the cortex where it facilitates synaptic formation and strengthening to encode the relevant linguistic information. This aspect of the mechanism is illustrated in Fig. 2.5. The whole model is assembled in Fig. 2.6.

THE EVIDENCE

What evidence do we have that this mechanism operates in second language acquisition. At the outset, it must be stated that we have no *direct* evidence. There is no neurobiological research that shows activity or changes in the amygdala, orbitofrontal cortex, body proper, or basal ganglia related to SLA. However, second language learners have brains, and we know brains make appraisals and generate foraging; so where we see appraisals and intellectual foraging influencing SLA, we can hypothesize that the neural mechanisms described in this chapter are involved. Evidence for the role of stimulus appraisal and mental foraging in SLA can be found in autobiographies of second language learners.

Language Learner Autobiographies

Language-learner autobiographies provide a retrospective longitudinal view of the influence of stimulus appraisal and behavioral and mental foraging on

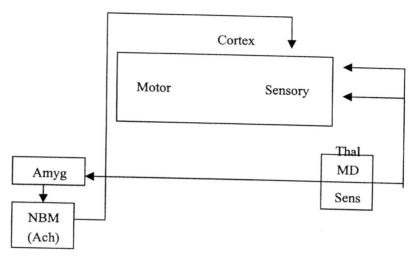

FIG. 2.5. The mechanism for laying down memories for language items encountered in learning.
NBM = Nucleus basalis of Meynert
Ach = Acetylcholine
Thal = Thalamus
Sens = Sensory thalamus

SLA. Sources of such autobiographical data come from personal histories of language acquisition elicited from learners and from spontaneous histories published by authors describing their language-learning experiences (Schumann, 1997). To illustrate the role of appraisal and foraging in SLA, we summarize the autobiography of Barbara Hilding presented in Schumann (1997). Barbara's first language was English, but she spent a good deal of time as a child with her Ukrainian speaking grandparents and acquired that language as well. She studied French in elementary and high school (grades 6-12), and recalled that the instruction was poor, and it appeared that the teachers frequently did not know French very well. More importantly, she noted that the acquisition of French was not a relevant goal, and there was no expectation by her family or community that she or her peers would learn the language. Thus, on the dimensions of goal relevance and self and social compatibility, the language-learning situation did not generate positive appraisals. It appears that the French classes were simply routine and largely irrelevant school tasks. She commented, "As ... [French] had no connection with my life, I was not moti-

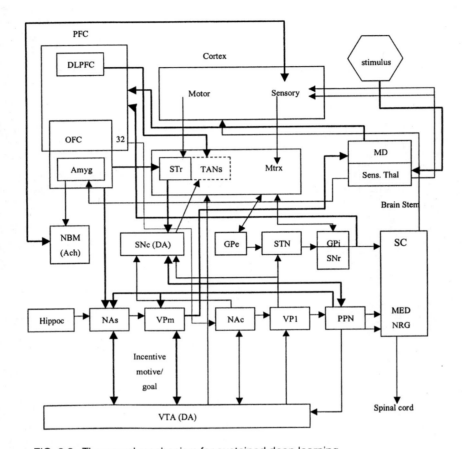

FIG. 2.6. The neural mechanism for sustained deep learning.
DLPFC = Dorsolateral prefrontal cortex
GPe = Globus pallidus, external segment
STN = Subthalamic nucleus
GPi = Globus pallidus, internal segment
SNr = substantia nigra, pars reticulata
SC = superior colliculus

vated to learn the language" (p. 160). When Barbara entered college she enrolled in a first-year French course but dropped out shortly afterward.

Ten years later, when she would have been 27 or 28 years old and was working as a letter carrier, she developed a romantic relationship with a French Canadian. She then became motivated to learn French in order to speak her

boyfriend's language, to interact with his family and friends, and to participate in his culture. Learning French was now a relevant goal and because her job afforded her ample free time, her coping potential was substantial. Then Barbara began to forage for knowledge about French and for skill in using French. She enrolled in a first semester French class at a local university. She spent 4 to 6 hours a day working in the language laboratory. She took every opportunity to learn. Before going grocery shopping, she would make a list of everything she wanted to buy and would rehearse the pronunciation of the items with her French-speaking partner until she could pronounce them perfectly. Barbara did so well in her first semester French course that she was advanced directly into 5th/6th semester French. It became apparent that her appraisals on the coping dimension had two aspects: she had the time to devote to the task, and she also had considerable talent. Barbara foraged with great intensity. She spent many hours each night doing French homework. When she found segments of language on a tape that she did not understand, she played them over and over again. She read dictionaries and studied verb lists. She also got up early in the morning to have breakfast ready for her boyfriend so that he could review her homework with her. In the first summer after undertaking the study of French, Barbara expanded her foraging space by going to Quebec to study in a 6 week immersion program. Her success generated positive appraisals in terms of her self and social image, and discovering that she was capable learner, she made positive appraisals of the language learning enterprise in terms of her ability to cope. Thus, for her, language learning became enjoyable and was also appraised positively in terms of pleasantness.

Barbara noted that the positive appraisal of her French Canadian boyfriend led to a positive appraisal of learning French (amplified by her aptitude for it), and these appraisals also led to interest in and a valorization of French literature, cinema, music, people, and the structure of both standard French and French dialects. This extension demonstrates the associative nature of the appraisal process. The positive (or negative) assessment of an agent, action, or object is likely to lead to a similar appraisal of related people, events, and things. Barbara's relationship with her boyfriend eventually ended, but her passion for French continued. When she had completed a sufficient number of credits in French, she spent a summer in a language program in Avignon, France. When she returned, she entered graduate school and became a teaching assistant. This employment motivated further mental foraging as she spent several hours preparing for each class she taught. This intellectual effort achieved two goals. It made her teaching effective and vastly improved her knowledge and skill in French. In graduate school, Barbara was recognized as a talented student and teacher. She won fellowships and awards, received her graduate degree, achieved near native proficiency, and became a university teacher of that language. She continues her foraging/learning by spending most summers in francophone areas of the world.

Later she also undertook the study of Spanish. She and a friend planned a trip to Mexico. Before leaving, she worked with a set of records containing Spanish lessons and acquired some basic knowledge of the language. Her experience in Mexico was very positive. She enjoyed the people, the language, and the culture. Not surprisingly, given her experience with French, she did quite well learning the language. When she returned to Canada, she took a first-year Spanish class, did well and went to a second-year course. She reports that in the second year, the work became more difficult (she mentions the irregular verbs), but more importantly, she saw that she was not likely to have the opportunity to use Spanish in the future and the learning lost its goal relevance. The pleasant memories of her visit to Mexico failed to sustain her motivation and she stopped studying the language. This experience illustrates that in spite of initial positive appraisals in terms of coping potential, self and social compatibility, and pleasantness, when the appraisal of goal relevance became negative, efforts (i.e., foraging) to learn ceased.

Later Barbara also studied German. She made very positive appraisals of her first year German class. She was impressed with her teacher's competence and the organized manner in which she taught the course. She appreciated and responded to the teacher's high expectations. (This was not true for all students. The class began with 35 enrollees and by the end of the first week, when it became clear what would be demanded of them, only 12 remained.) Barbara made excellent progress, and in the following year enrolled in second year German. Fourteen of the 19 students in this class were native speakers of the language. She found she could not participate; she could not formulate the responses quickly enough. She was intimidated, felt inadequate, and eventually began to skip class. After the course was over (although she received an excellent grade), she abandoned the study of German. In first-year German, Barbara had made positive appraisals of the learning situation in terms of goal relevance, coping ability, self and social image, and pleasantness. However, in the second year, when the situation was assessed negatively in terms of coping potential and self image, she finished the course but gave up the study of German.

It should be noted that Barbara provides her own control with respect to language learning aptitude, which we can assume was the same for all three languages but only resulted in high proficiency in one of them. Therefore, lack of aptitude was not an issue in her learning. Her experiences also speak to the critical period issue—she acquired near native proficiency in French in her late 20s and early 30s, well after what is assumed to be the close of the critical period.

Drugs of Abuse

Another source of evidence for the argument that the neural systems described in this chapter subserve motivation is the finding that dopamine, which plays such an important role in the motivational systems described, is also the neurotransmitter that appears to be affected by all drugs of abuse. We discussed how dopamine provides a reward signal when organisms encounter stimuli that predict the achievement of goals. That hit of dopamine is pleasurable. It is designed, as mentioned earlier, as a "go" signal to keep the foraging organism on task. Humans have cleverly figured out how to get that pleasurable hit independently of its biological function to guide goal directed activity. We have developed products that, when taken exogenously, affect the dopamine system and essentially co-opt it. This system that was designed by nature as a pleasurable predictor of reward, has become, with drugs of abuse, a straightforward nonfunctional source of pleasure. Next, we review how the various drugs of abuse operate on dopamine. The goal here is to understand that motivation is maintained by signals that predict reward in terms of the achievement of one's goal.

Alcohol is a depressant. Depressants in moderate use can lead to relaxation and lessening of inhibitions. They slow down brain processes and reduce fear. Depressants are often used to treat anxiety and insomnia (DuPont, 1997). Alcohol increases extracellular dopamine levels by stimulating dopaminergic cell firing (DiChiara, Acquas, Tanda, & Cadoni, 1993). Low doses of alcohol excite the VTA suggesting it provides a pharmacological "reward," which facilitates alcohol seeking (Gessa, Muntoni, Cullu, Vargiu, & Mereu, 1985). Alcohol, like most drugs of abuse, increases dopamine levels in the nucleus accumbens (DiChiara et al., 1993; Koob, 1997; Stolerman, 1993; Wise, 1996) compared to the dorsal caudate levels (DiChiara, 1995).

Cocaine, a psychomotor stimulant, has a potent effect on motor behavior. It has the ability to increase locomotion and cause stereotyped repetitive behaviors, tics and uncontrollable tremors (Hurd, 1996). Cocaine induces a wide range of affective states in humans, from an initial high (euphoria) to severe anxiety, paranoia, depression, and anhedonia. Cocaine promotes the increase of dopamine in synapses by blocking reuptake and thus leaving more dopamine in the synapse (DiChiara, 1995; DiChiara et al., 1993; DuPont, 1997).

Thus, dopamine cannot be retrieved effectively by axons in the brains of cocaine users; it accumulates in the synapses and produces euphoria, an exaggerated sense of well-being, and heightened feelings of energy (DuPont, 1997). It appears that the initiation of cocaine reward is controlled within the prefrontal cortex and perhaps the VTA (Bardo, 1998). The mediation of cocaine reward seems to reside in the nucleus accumbens (Ikemoto & Panksepp, 1999). Amphetamine stimulates dopamine producing cells by releasing dopamine through an impulse independent cocaine sensitive carrier mechanism (DiChiara & Imperato, 1988; DiChiara et al., 1993). With amphetamine drugs, activation of the reward circuitry occurs within the nucleus accumbens. Microinjections of amphetamine into the nucleus accumbens assists responding to stimulation in the VTA (Huston-Lyons & Kornetsky, 1992). Solid evidence, found through amphetamine self-administration and conditioned place preference testing paradigms, has also shown that the nucleus accumbens has a role in the initiation and the mediation of amphetamine reward (Bardo, 1998). In the nucleus accumbens shell, dopamine aids the formation of new incentive relationships to environmental cues and contexts in which drug taking occurs (Ikemoto et al., 1999).

Opiates such as heroin also work primarily by blocking the reuptake of naturally occurring neurotransmitters (DuPont, 1997). Along with other drugs of abuse, opiates increase dopamine concentrations in mesolimbic and nigrostriatal pathways (DiChiara & Imperato, 1988). Most opiate research shows that dopamine levels increase more in the mesolimbic pathway at the level of the VTA (Huston-Lyons & Kornetsky, 1992) than in the nigrostriatal pathways. Acute administration of the opiate, morphine, increases dopamine in the nucleus accumbens with smaller dopamine increases in the striatum (DiChiara & Imperato, 1988; Wood & Altar, 1988; Wood & Richard, 1982).

Several perceived psychopharmacological effects of nicotine include increased subjective arousal, sedation/relaxation, and appetite suppression (Clarke, 1991). Nicotine is considerably less stimulating than alcohol, amphetamine, cocaine, and heroin (Warburton, 1991). Dopamine, agonized by nicotine, is released from the same cells of the VTA and the nucleus accumbens as are drugs as diverse as heroin, alcohol, and cocaine, although it operates by an entirely unique mechanism. Nicotine receptors, situated on the dopamine neuron itself, elevate nucleus accumbens dopamine levels by directly stimulating dopaminergic cell firing (Wise, 1996). Nicotine excites the VTA neurons apparently via direct depolarizing action on the host dopaminergic cells themselves (Corrigal, 1991). Like amphetamine's dependence on mesolimbic dopamine, nicotine (with certain qualifications) produces similar locomotor stimulation, reinforcing effects, and the ability to enhance the rewarding effect of electrical brain stimulation (Clarke, 1991).

These findings on the relationship between dopamine and reward, along with the earlier discussion of how dopamine operates through the appraisal of environmental stimuli in relation to their rewarding qualities, show how motivation in second language learning is simply the appraisal of stimuli as positive or negative in relation to the goal of acquiring the language. If the appraisals are positive, the learner will undertake action to acquire the language; if negative, action tendencies toward stimuli associated with the target language will be diminished.

IMPLICATIONS

We suggest that perhaps the major implications deriving from the theory and research that we have reported is that stimulus appraisal may be the common denominator in various types of motivation. Motivations appear to be patterns of stimulus appraisal. A limited number of appraisal dimensions (such as the 5 indicated by Scherer: novelty, pleasantness, goal relevance, coping potential, and self and social compatibility) can pattern in various ways to constitute motivations. For example, Gardner (1985) in his explorations of attitude and motivation in SLA focused mainly on appraisals of pleasantness in relation to the goal of language learning; Clement, Dornyei, and Noels (1994) focused on goal relevance and pleasantness. Schmidt and Savage (1992) investigating Csikszentmihalyi's (Csikszentmihalyi & Larson, 1987) notion of intrinsic motivation examined primarily appraisals of coping potential and secondarily appraisals of goal relevance and self and social compatibility. Schmidt, Boraie, and Kassabgy (1996) investigating value expectancy theories of motivation elicited in their questionnaire appraisals of goal relevance, pleasantness, and coping potential. To the extent that motivation directs SLA, at a more basic level, it is guided by stimulus appraisal which is implemented by the amygdala and orbitofrontal cortex and which is supported by dopaminergic activity in the basal ganglia.

It would appear that evolution has provided us with a biological appraisal system which operates along a limited set of dimensions to determine the motivational relevance of stimuli. Why might this be the case? In a simplified way, the brain can be seen as implementing the integration of three systems: a posterior sensory system, an anterior motor system, and a more or less ventral appraisal system that allows an individual to choose appropriate motor and/or mental behavior in relation to the survival and thrival relevance of the sensory

stimuli. Such a system makes the individual adaptable to changing present circumstances. The more flexible the appraisal system is, the better the organism
will adapt and thrive (Schumann, 1997).

However, appraisal systems are not infinitely flexible. As discussed earlier, they operate on the basis of stored memories about past encounters with
the same or similar stimuli. But everyone's experience is limited, and therefore, stimulus situations will be encountered in which the organism may not
be able to make appropriate appraisals. At the same time, individuals may
have had certain powerful emotional experiences (perhaps early in life) that
strongly bias their appraisal systems to interpret certain stimulus situations
in stereotypical ways. When the match is good, motor and mental action will
be appropriate, but when the stereotype is overgeneralized the appraisals
may be maladaptive.

What does this say about the kind of motivation that is best for SLA? In the
past, the debate was between instrumental and integrative motivation. Recent
investigations have examined the effectiveness of intrinsic motivation and
value-expectancy motives. Based on the language learner autobiography presented here and those in Schumann (1997), we argue that there may not be a
best motivation. What seems to be necessary is sufficient positive appraisals
along one or more of the five dimensions suggested to sustain the effort for the
5 to 8 years necessary to learn the second language well. The best motivation
will be any pattern or patterns of appraisal that will sustain learning until proficiency is achieved.

3   The Neurobiology of Procedural Memory

Namhee Lee

INTRODUCTION

As second/foreign-language learning proceeds, the second/foreign language speaker comes to use the morphosyntax and phonology of the target language more automatically, that is, with less and less inner rehearsal, preparation, or conscious effort. This chapter argues that acquiring this automaticity, with regard to the rule-related aspects of an L2, involves proceduralization of the linguistic information of the target language through neural structures that are embedded deep in the brain, collectively referred to as the basal ganglia (BG).

Some researchers who follow Chomskian Universal Grammar theory may argue that the automatization is a natural process that proceeds as the innate "grammar module" is activated when the learner is exposed to the environment of the target language. This chapter, in contrast, argues that at least with respect to second language acquisition, automatization is not a function of an innate grammar, but a process that occurs through a domain-general learning mechanism in the brain that is used not only for language but also for motor and other cognitive skill learning.

Investigating the BG to understand linguistic functions is not what neurolinguists usually do. In 1861, Pierre Paul Broca reported that his aphasic patients had localized lesions in the frontal cortex. Several years later, Karl Wernicke presented another kind of aphasia that stemmed from lesions in the posterior part of the superior temporal gyrus. Since these reports, most neurolinguistic studies have tried to explain language by focusing on those areas of the neocortex. However, the neocortical areas are not self-sufficient or autonomous entities. They are massively connected to other subcortical brain structures, all of which cooperate to perform diverse functions. A comprehensive consideration of the anatomy and physiology of the whole brain is necessary in order to have a more complete picture of language and its acquisition.

DEFINITION OF PROCEDURAL MEMORY
AND AUTOMATIZATION

Automatization is another name for acquiring procedural memory. As illustrated in the introduction to this book, the human memory system has short-term memory (working memory included) and long-term memory components. Long-term memory is again classified into two categories: declarative or explicit memory and nondeclarative or implicit memory. Explicit/declarative memory (DM) is again subclassified into semantic memory and episodic memory. Implicit or nondeclarative memory (NDM) is subclassified to conditioning, priming, and procedural memory, which is the topic of this chapter.

Fabbro (1999) asserted that procedural memory is concerned with the learning of motor and cognitive procedures through not only highly developed cerebral structures but also subcortical structures such as the basal ganglia and cerebellum. One acquires this type of memory through the repeated execution of a task. Normally, one is not aware of the nature of the knowledge, and sometimes does not remember when and how the skill was learned. This memory is used, for example, when one learns how to play a musical instrument, how to dance, how to play a sport, or how to speak native language.

Numerous activities in our daily lives are learned and performed procedurally, that is, automatically and unconsciously. When a professional pianist plays Beethoven, he or she is not aware of the position or the movement of the fingers. While she watches the score of the music, his or her fingers, hands, and feet fly freely, automatically, and unconsciously. Likewise, when one speaks in native language, one does not consciously move the oral articulatory organs. People are oblivious to the grammar rules that were learned in school. One does not pay attention to the phonological rules that govern the pronunciation of his or her speech. Talking flows freely, automatically, and unconsciously. These are automatic, or proceduralized, motor and cognitive behaviors. Without this automaticity, humans, and any entity in the animal kingdom for this matter, would not be able to survive simply because the cognitive demands would be too taxing (Graybiel, 1998).

BRAIN STRUCTURES INVOLVED IN PROCEDURAL LEARNING

Hikosaka and his colleagues studied the neural substrates for motor sequence learning as a prototypical example of procedural learning, and their work has revealed the neural mechanism for this process. They developed a series of experiments using common Japanese monkeys (Macaca fuscata) and human subjects (Hikosaka, Miyashita, Miyachi, Sakai, & Lu, 1998; Hikosaka, Rand, Miyachi, & Miyashita, 1995; Hikosaka et al., 1996, 1999; Kawagoe, Takikawa, & Hikosaka, 1998; Nakamura, Sakai, & Hikosaka, 1999; Rand, Hikosaka, Miyachi, Lu, & Miyashita, 1998; Sakai, Hikosaka, Miyauchi, Sasaki, & Putz, 1998; Sakai et al., 2000). In their monkey experiments, the subjects learn, by pure trial and error, the order of ten buttons that should be pushed sequentially. With repetitive practice, the monkeys acquire the motor skills necessary to accomplish this task, error-free.

Hikosaka and his colleagues examined such learning with fMRI imaging (Hikosaka et al., 1995, 1998, 1999; Sakai et al., 1998, 2000), muscimal (a GABA agonist) injection experiments (Hikosaka et al., 1998; Nakamura et al., 1999), and behavioral observation (Rand et al., 1998). All their research confirmed that during the early stages of learning, the presupplementary motor cortex and the anterior part of the basal ganglia (i.e., the head of the caudate nucleus) are recruited to initiate sequence learning. After the sequence is overlearned and automatized, the cerebellar dentate nucleus and the posterior part of the basal ganglia (the middle and posterior part of the putamen) are recruited to store and retrieve the procedural memory. Table 3.1 summarizes the results of their experiments.

These findings are further supported by Graybiel (1998). According to Graybiel, when new learning takes place, the anterior striatum (caudate nucleus), anterior PFC, and anterior cingulate are recruited because these anterior structures work to support attention. When a learned sequence is performed, the putamen, premotor, and motor cortex are enlisted (Graybiel, 1998; Kimura & Graybiel, 1995). Therefore, Hikosaka and his team and Graybiel and her col-

TABLE 3.1
Activated Brain Areas in Initial and Advanced
Stages of Sequence Learning

Stages of learning	Brain areas involved	
	Cortex	Basal ganglia and others
Early stage (learning)	Presupplementary motor area	Head of the caudate nucleus
Overlearned stage (storing and retrieving)		Middle and posterior putamen, dentate nucleus of the cerebellum

leagues have shown that the basal ganglia is involved in learning, storing and retrieving procedural memories. This research shows what the motor mechanisms do automatically when external sensory or internal cognitive stimuli are presented. As learning proceeds, the association between the motor activity and the stimulus becomes strengthened and automatized accordingly.

BASAL GANGLIA'S CONTRIBUTIONS TO LEARNING

The previous section argued that the basal ganglia is involved in automatization. The following sections describe the structure of the basal ganglia, the general anatomy and physiology of the basal ganglia, the neuronal connections involved in chunking, the connections from the basal ganglia to the thalamus, and connections from the cortex to the basal ganglia to thalamus and back to the cortex.

Anatomy and Physiology

Table 3.2 and Fig. 3.1 present the structure of the BG. The BG is composed of the dorsal BG (also called dorsal striatum), the ventral striatum and the ven-

TABLE 3.2
Structure of the BG

	Striatal Complex	Pallidal Complex
Dorsal Basal Ganglia (Striatum)	Neostriatum (Striatum): Caudate Nucleus & Putamen	Paleostratum (Pallidum): Globus Pallidus (Internal and External Segments)
Ventral Striatum	Nucleus Acumbens & Olafactory Tubercle	
Ventral Pallidum		Substantia Innominata

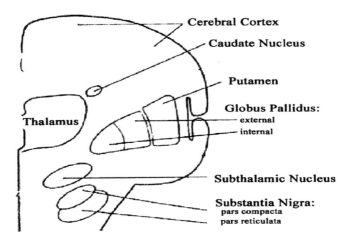

FIG. 3.1. Anatomy of the Basal ganglia.

tral pallidum. The dorsal BG is the core structure, and is classified into the neostriatum, or simply striatum (Parent, 1996), which consists of the caudate nucleus and putamen, and the paleostriatum, or simply pallidum, which is the globus pallidus and is composed of internal and external segments. The ventral striatum includes the nucleus accumbens and the olfactory tubercle. The ventral pallidum is the substantia innominata. Each part of the basal ganglia has associated areas it communicates with. The dorsal striatum is associated with the substantia nigra, the subthalamic nucleus, and the parabrachial pontine reticular formation. The ventral striatum is associated with the amygdala and the ventral tegmental area. The associated areas are reciprocally connected with the basal ganglia through closed loops, which are typical of basal ganglia circuitry. These associated areas exert a profound modulatory influence on the basal ganglia (Ma, 1997; Parent, 1996).

Another way of classifying the BG is by dividing it into the striatal complex, which is so named because of striating of traversing fibers (the middle column in Table 3.2), and the pallidal complex (the right column in Table 3.2), which looks pale. The striatal complex consists of the neostriatum (the caudate nucleus and the putamen) and the ventral striatum (the nucleus accumbens and the olfactory tubercle). At the cellular level, the neostriatum is composed of the striosomes, or patches, and the matrisomes, or matrix (Parent, 1996). There are two types of neurons in the neostriatum:

spiny neurons and aspiny neurons. The former have spiny dendrites and long axons, and constitute the projection neurons that receive massive afferents from all areas of the cerebral cortex (Graybiel, 1998) except from the primary visual and primary auditory cortices (Purves, 1997). The spiny neurons also project to structures such as the pallidum and the substantia nigra. The neurons of the neostriatum are largely GABAergic, which is the major inhibitory neurotransmitter of the central nervous system (Purves, 1997). Therefore, when they are activated, they directly inhibit and modulate their targets. The aspiny neurons have smooth dendrites and short axons. TANs (tonically active neurons) are aspiny interneurons modulating local activity within the neostriatum. As indicated in chapter 2, these structures are also involved in motivation.

The pallidal complex is composed of the paleostriatum (internal and external segments of the globus pallidus (GPi and GPe, respectively) and the ventral pallidum (the substantia innominata). The main afferent input to the globus pallidus is from the striatal complex. The GPi projects to the thalamus, and the GPe projects to the subthalamic nucleus (STN), which, in turn, projects to GPi. The pallidum also contains primarily GABAergic neurons with high rates of spontaneous activity, and therefore they tonically inhibit their target neurons.

Although the STN is not a part of the BG, it is critically involved in the BG loops. The neurons of the STN are inactive under normal conditions because of the constant inhibition from the GPe. But when the inhibition from the GPe is removed, the STN cells become highly active and excite the target neurons in the GPi with the excitatory neurotransmitter, glutamate.

Other structures critically participating in the BG loops are the substantia nigra pars compacta (SNc), substantia nigra pars reticulata (SNr), and the ventral tegmental area (VTA). The SNc projects mainly to the neostriatum, using dopamine as a transmitter. Dopamine excites or inhibits the target neurons depending on the type of receptors on the postsynaptic membrane. The SNr projects mainly to the thalamus, tonically inhibiting the target neurons. The VTA forms reciprocal loops with ventral striatum (the nucleus accumbens and olfactory tubercle), the amygdala, and other limbic structures, using dopaminergic neurons.

Convergence, Divergence, and Reconvergence

The projection patterns of the basal ganglia involve convergence, divergence, and reconvergence. The neurons of the neostriatum, mainly medium spiny neurons, receive massive inputs from all areas of the cerebral cortex. These inputs take two forms: convergence and divergence. In convergence, inputs from functionally related multiple areas in the neocortex tend to converge on the neurons of the striatum selectively and precisely. About 10,000 neurons from the neocortex converge on a single projection neuron of the striatum (Graybiel, 1998; Joel & Weiner, 1998). In other words, 10,000 pieces of functionally related cortical information project to and are synthesized on one striatal neuron.

In divergence, inputs from a small site of the neocortex tend to be widely distributed in the striatum. These distributed inputs form partially interconnected clusters through the striatal interneurons (TANs). During learning, these striatal interneurons acquire conditioned responses gradually by encoding stimulus-response patterns in the striatal projection neurons that they influence. Systems of these input modules of convergence and divergence serve as templates for building new associations in the striatum, selecting which inputs result in output activation, and shaping corticostriatal remapping (Graybiel, 1998). On the other hand, reconvergence means that the functionally related striatal neurons project to functionally related target neurons in the globus pallidus or the Snr.

Through the three projection patterns above, cortical information is sorted and synthesized through the basal ganglia circuits. This information sorting is referred to as *chunking* by Graybiel (1998). According to Graybiel, cortical areas and the striatum cooperate and gradually form codes for movement sequences with specific temporal and spatial orders. This gradual tuning of modular populations of neurons in the striatum, the spatiotemporal binding of the striatal neurons by TANs, and the reconvergence of the information onto striatal output targets are the mechanisms that bring about chunking (Graybiel, 1998). Through chunking, motor and cognitive action sequences are formed as routines that can be subsequently executed as performance units. This chunking process is a mechanism for the learning and expression of motor and cognitive action repertoires.

The chunking process is modulated by the dopaminergic system. The striosomes of the striatum receive massive input from the prefrontal cortex (PFC), especially from the anterior cingulate, medial PFC, and caudal orbitofrontal cortex (OFC). These regions are connected to the amygdala, and their neurons fire to signal upcoming rewarding situations or lack of reward (see chap. 2 of this book). Striosomes are also reciprocally connected to the dopamine-containing neurons of the substantia nigra pars compacta (SNc), which respond to salient attention-attracting stimuli and to conditioned stimuli predictive of future rewards (Kawagoe et al., 1998). Therefore, the status of the dopaminergic system affects the efficacy of the chunking mechanism.

In terms of cellular level alterations, the following is an example of what changes take place in the striatal neurons during convergence. The membrane potentials of the projection neurons of the striatum fluctuate between a down-state and an up-state, depending on the intensity of the cortical input. These neurons generate few spontaneous action potentials (see chap. 4 of this book for more detailed explanation of action potential system), so they require strong input from afferent fibers in order to be activated (Graybiel, 1998; Purves, 1997). In the absence of strong cortical input, the striatal projection neurons do not generate action potentials, that is, they remain in a down-state. When there is a strong and temporally coherent input from the cortex, action potentials are generated in the striatal neurons, creating an up-state (Graybiel, 1998). Graybiel reported,

> The cortical inputs are glutamatergic, and the projection neurons have both non-NMDA and NMDA receptors. When they are in down-state, NMDA receptors are blocked, and glutamate acts through AMPA/kainate receptors. Under conditions of strong and temporally coherent activation, driving the neurons into up-state, NMDA receptors begin to become active with further inputs, promoting longer postsynaptic response times to favor input summation and also favoring NMDA-receptor mediated forms of plasticity. (Graybiel, 1998, p. 120)

Figure 3.2 schematically illustrates how convergence, divergence, and re-convergence work to bring about cellular change in the striatum. If function-ally related cortical areas 1, 2, and 3 project to striatal cell A, these convergent projections promote the up-state of neuron A, which causes it to

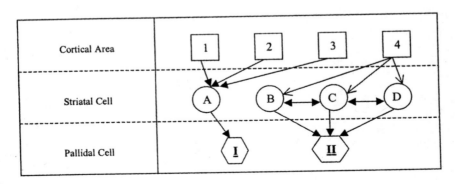

FIG. 3.2. Convergence, divergence, and reconvergence.

fire. This, in turn, leads to more activation of NMDA receptors in A, which then more readily causes long term potentiation in that neuron (see chap. 4). If coherent and repetitive cortical activation on neuron A occurs, then long-term change in this cell gradually takes place (Graybiel, 1998). If cortical area 4 projects to striatal neurons B, C, and D, then these divergent projections are interconnected by striatal interneurons (marked by bidirectional arrows in the figure). Striatal neurons B, C, and D reconverge onto the neuron in the output target, pallidal cell II, in the globus pallidus or in the SNr.

Projections from cortical areas 1, 2, and 3 illustrate convergence. Projections from 4 to striatal cells B, C, and D represents divergence, and the striatal projections to pallidal cell II shows reconvergence.

Direct Pathway and Indirect Pathway

Simply speaking, cortical inputs pass through the BG system, go on to the thalamus, and return to the cortical areas, forming a loop. However, inside the BG, each loop diverges into two pathways: the direct pathway (DP) and the indirect pathway (IP). These two pathways create a balance in the inhibitory flow of the BG, and function by modulating the extent of the inhibition on target nuclei. Generally speaking, the DP facilitates the flow of information through the thalamus, that is, the DP increases the activity of the thalamus and the consequent excitation of the cerebral cortex. On the other hand, the IP inhibits the flow of information through the thalamus. That is, the IP decreases the activity of the thalamus and consequently decreases the activity of the cerebral cortex.

Direct Pathway (DP)

Table 3.3 summarizes the steps of the DP, and they are schematically presented in Fig. 3.3. In Fig. 3.3, the pathway form the cortex, to the striatum, to the internal segment of the globus pallidus (GPi), to the thalamus, and back to the cortex is the DP. The following explanation is complex, but the system is important for subsquent discussion of the striatum:

1. From the cortex to the striatum:
   As mentioned in the preceding section, the medium spiny neurons of the striatum receive extensive projections from diverse areas of the neocortex. The afferent projections from the cerebral cortex use the excitatory glutamatergic system; therefore, they excite the tar-

TABLE 3.3
Direct Pathway

	Neocortex →	Matrisome of the Striatum →	Gpi and SNr →	Thalamus →	Neocortex →
Characteristics of the neurons	Excitatory (Glutamate)	Phasically Inhibitory (GABA)	Tonically inhibitory (GABA)	Tonically excitatory (Glutamate)	
State of the neurons as the result of the influence from the previous step		Excited	Inhibited	Excited	Excited
Influence to the next step	Excite the next	Inhibit the next	Cannot inhibit the next	Excite the next	

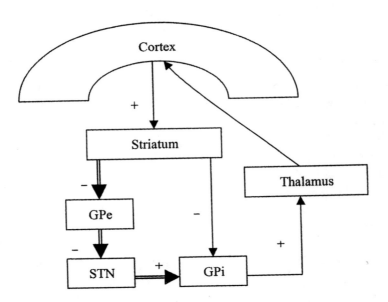

FIG. 3.3. Direct and indirect pathways.
GPe: globus pallidus external segment; GPi: globus pallidus internal segment; STN: subthalamic nucleus; +: activation; –: inhibition
The pathway marked by double line arrows is the indirect pathway, and the single line arrows mark the direct pathway.

get medium spiny neurons in the striatum, which have little or no spontaneous activity (Purves, 1997).

2. From the striatum to GPi and Substantia nigra pars reticulata (Snr): The medium spiny neurons of the striatum are phasically active only when they are excited by cortical inputs; they are not spontaneously active. The efferent neurons of the striatum mainly use GABA; thus, when they are active, they inhibit the target neurons in the GPi and SNr.

3. From the GPi and SNr to the thalamus: The next step in the DP is from the GPi and the SNr to the thalamus. The neurons in the GPi and SNr have a high rate of spontaneous inhibition; thus, when there is no inhibitory input from the striatum, they tonically inhibit the target neurons in the thalamus. If the GPi and the SNr receive inhibitory inputs from the striatum, the neurons of the GPi and SNr are inhibited, and thus cannot inhibit the target neurons in the thalamus. Thus, the thalamus neurons are disinhibited (i.e., activated).

4. From the thalamus to the cortex: The final step in the DP is from the thalamus to the cortex. The thalamic neurons are glutamatergic and tonically excite the target neurons. When inhibited by the inhibitory neurons of the striatum, the inhibitory neurons of the GPi and SNr become inactive, and thus cannot inhibit the thalamic neurons. Disinhibited thalamus neurons are spontaneously active and excite the cerebral cortex.

Indirect Pathway (IP)

The indirect pathway goes from the striatum to the GPe, to the subthalamic nucleus (STN), to the GPi, to the thalamus, and then to the neocortex. The flow of the IP is pictured in Fig. 3.3 (the double line arrows) and in Table 3.4, and is described in the following steps.

1. From the cortex to the striatum: same as the DP.

2. From the striatum to the Gpe: The striatum projects to the GPe, instead of the GPi. The cells of the striatum are inhibitory. Therefore, when they are activated, they inhibit GPe.

3. From GPe to STN: Like the GPi, GPe cells also use the GABAergic system, and have a high spontaneous firing rate. The efferent neurons from the GPe tonically inhibit the neurons of the STN. If the striatum cells are ac-

TABLE 3.4
Indirect Pathway

	Neo-cortex →	Matrisome of the Striatum →	GPe →	STN →	Gpi and SNr →	Thalamus →	Neo-cortex
Characteristics of the cells	Excitatory	Phasically Inhibitory	Tonically inhibitory	Tonically excitatory	Tonically inhibitory	Tonically excitatory	
State of the neurons as the result of the influence from the previous step		Excited	Inhibited	Not inhibited	Excited	Inhibited	Not excited
Influence to the next step	Excite the next	Inhibit the next	Cannot inhibit the next	Excite the next	Inhibit the next	Cannot excite the next	Not excited

tive, they inhibit the GPe, and then the neurons of the GPe are inhibited and cannot inhibit the target neurons of the STN. Thus, the neurons of the STN become active.

4. From STN to Gpi:
   The neurons of the STN are glutamatergic. They are spontaneously active when there is no inhibition from the GPe. Like the glutamatergic projections of the cerebral cortex, the neurons of the STN are excitatory and excite the target neurons in the GPi.
5. From GPi to the thalamus: same as the DP.
   The neurons of the GPi are spontaneously active and tonically inhibitory, thus, they inhibit the target neurons of the thalamus when they excited by the neurons of the STN.
6. From the thalamus to the cortex: the same as DP.
   When inhibited by the neurons of the GPi, the neurons of the thalamus cannot excite the target neurons of the cortex.

Parallel Circuits in the Basal Ganglia

There are five parallel circuits in the BG, and each circuit has its own DP and IP. Each circuit connects distinct cortical areas and distinct striatal areas, and has a distinct function. These circuits are called *closed circuits*. The closed circuits are defined as striato-cortical pathways that project back to the cortical areas where the pathways originate (Joel & Weiner, 1998). The closed circuits are interconnected and directly influence each other. This cross-circuit influence takes place through open components (Ma, 1997), or *open pathways* (Joel & Weiner, 1998). The open pathways are striatocortical pathways that terminate in cortical areas that are different from the cortical area in which the pathway originated (Joel & Weiner, 1998). In other words, the closed circuits are units for distinct functions and the open pathways are the routes by which each closed circuit influences other closed circuits.

Closed Circuits

Ma (1997) presented five cortical-basal ganglia loops: the motor loop, the oculomotor loop, the dorsolateral prefrontal loop, the lateral orbitofrontal loop, and the limbic loop. Joel and Weiner (1998) referred to the motor loop as the motor split circuit, the dorsolateral prefrontal loop and lateral orbitofrontal loop as the associative split circuit, and the last as the limbic circuit. Each circuit originates in functionally different regions of the cerebral cortices, passes through distinct regions of the striatum, innervates distinct parts of the pallidum, modulates different areas of the thalamus, and returns to the cortical regions in which it originated. Each loop is explained next and summarized in Table 3.5.

The *motor loop* is involved in somatosensory and somatic motor control (Ma, 1997) or sensorimotor aspects of behavior (Parent, 1996). This loop originates in the supplementary motor area (SMA), premotor area, and motor cortex, and passes through the putamen (Ma, 1997). The putamen also receives input from the primary and secondary somatosensory cortices in the parietal lobe, the secondary visual cortices in the occipital lobe, and the auditory association area in the temporal lobe (Purves, 1997). Then, the loop diverges into the DP and the IP in distinct parts of the pallidum, innervates distinct part of the thalamus, and finally comes back to the same cortical areas. As learning or automatization advances, the motor circuit can perform well-learned motor sequences without help from the associative circuit. This circuit, thus, selects and executes simple and specific motor acts.

The *occulomotor loop* controls orientation and gaze. This loop originates in the frontal eye field, dorsolateral prefrontal cortex, and posterior parietal cortex. It passes through the body of the caudate nucleus, the DP or the IP, the thalamus, and finally returns to the original cortical areas.

The *dorsolateral prefrontal loop* originates in the dorsolateral prefrontal cortex, posterior parietal cortex, and premotor area. It passes through the dorsolateral part of the head of the caudate nucleus, the DP or the IP, the

TABLE 3.5
Closed Circuits: Functions and Involved Structures

	Functions	Originating cortical areas	Striatum	Pallidum	Thalamus
Motor	Somato sensory and somatic motor control	SMA, motor, premotor, primary and secondary somatosensory, secondary visual, auditory association	Putamen	Gpi (ventral portion), Snr (dorsolateral portion)	Ventral lateral nucleus (oral part), ventral anterior nucleus, centromedian nucleus
Occulomotor	Orientation and gaze	Frontal eye field, dorsolateral PFC, posterior parietal	Caudate (body)	Gpi (central portion), Snr (ventrolateral portion)	Ventral anterior nucleus (magnocellular part), medial dorsal nucleus
Dorsolateral PFC	Cognitive process	Dorsolateral PFC, premotor, posterior parietal	Head of caudate (dorsolateral part)	Gpi (lateral portion), Snr (ventromedial portion)	Ventral anterior nucleus (parvocellular part), medial dorsal nucleus (parvocellular part)
Lateral orbitofrontal	Cognitive process	Orbitofrontal, superior and inferior temporal	Head of caudate (ventromedial part)	Gpi (medial portion), Snr (dorsomedial portion)	Ventral anterior nucleus (magnocellular part), medial dorsal nucleus (magnocellular part)
Limbic	Emotional and visceral functions and motivation	Anterior cingulate, hippocampal complex, entorhinal cortex, superior and inferior temporal gyri	Ventral striatum	Ventral pallidum, ventral tegmental area	Medial dorsal nucleus (parvocellular part)

thalamus, and again terminates in the originating cortical areas. The *lateral orbitofrontal loop* originates in the lateral orbitofrontal cortex, superior and inferior temporal gyri, and anterior cingulate. It passes through the ventromedial part of the head of the caudate nucleus, the DP or the IP, the thalamus, and finally goes to the originating cortical areas.

Generally speaking, the third and the fourth loops can be called the *associative circuit* (Joel & Weiner, 1998; Purves, 1997). They originate mainly in the multimodal association cortical areas, which process not just one type of sensory information but rather synthesize multiple external sensory and internal cognitive stimuli. This circuit is active when one is consciously processing complex cognitive aspects of behavior such as planning, scheming, temporal, and spatial sequencing. That is, the associative circuit selects and executes motor programs and steps, which are broader and less specific schemes of movement (Joel & Weiner, 1998; Ma, 1997; Parent, 1996; Purves, 1997).

The *limbic loop* is involved in motivational and emotional and visceral functions. It originates in the anterior cingulate area, hippocampus, entorhinal cortex, and superior and inferior temporal gyri. This is the only circuit that passes through the ventral striatum (the olfactory tubercle and the nucleus accumbens) instead of the neostriatum. It is also the only circuit passing through the ventral pallidum (the substantia innominata) and ventral tegmental area (VTA) instead of GPi or SNr. This path finally projects to the medial dorsal nucleus of the thalamus and then returns to the cortical areas from which it originates.

The anatomical and functional differences among closed circuits explain why the head of the caudate nucleus is active in the initial stage of sequence learning and the middle and the posterior parts of the putamen are mobilized to process well-learned sequences. The head of the caudate nucleus participates in the dorsolateral PFC and lateral orbitofrontal closed circuits (associative circuits), and the putamen participates in the motor circuit. The head of the caudate nucleus of the associative circuits receives input from the prefrontal cortex, including orbitofrontal cortex, and premotor cortex among others. In contrast, the putamen receives input mainly from the premotor cortex, supplementary motor area, and primary motor cortex. The anterior part of the putamen is connected more closely to the premotor cortex, and its posterior part is connected more closely to the primary motor cortex.

Fuster (1996) noted that the dorsolateral frontal cortex is composed of three sub-divisions, which are hierarchically organized in terms of their functions. The most anterior part of it, the prefrontal cortex, is responsible for the highest and most global cognitive activities such as planning, developing broad schemes, and organizing time and spatial trajectories. Directly posterior to the PFC is the premotor area, including the supplementary motor cortex. This region takes care of intermediate-level plans and schemes, and attention (Fuster, 1996; Jueptner, Frith, Brooks, Frackowiak, & Passingham, 1997; Jueptner, Stephan et al., 1997). More posterior to the premotor area is the primary motor area, which is in charge of imminent actions that are concrete and specific (Fuster, 1996).

Based on the functional differences between the associative closed circuits and motor closed circuits and the difference among the cortical areas connected to those closed circuits, one can speculate that the head of the caudate nucleus participates in the learning process, because the learning process would need more global cognitive activity. In contrast, the more posterior part of the putamen is mobilized when a well-learned activity is performed, because execution of well-learned motor actions would not require much cognitive functioning such as planning or scheming.

Open Pathways

Each of the five closed circuits is modulated by input from other cortical centers through intrinsic BG connections, or the open pathways. Joel and Weiner (1998) described the construction and functions of the open components of the basal ganglia circuits. An open pathway is a striatocortical pathway that terminates in a cortical area that innervates a different striatal subregion. For example, the putamen, which receives input from the supplementary motor area, premotor area, primary motor cortex, and somato-sensory area, projects not only to the motor pallidum but also to the associative pallidum—the projections of which, in turn, arrive via the thalamus to the association cortices, such as the dorsolateral PFC, the OFC, and so on. Thus, the motor circuit can influence the association cortices. Likewise, the caudate nucleus, which receives projections from the association cortices, also projects to the motor pallidum, the processes of which finally reach the motor cortex via the thalamus, in addition to the associative pallidum and the association cortex. These crossings seem to take place among all the circuits. The motor part of the striatum can influence the association and the limbic cortex, the associative part of the striatum can influence the motor and limbic cortex, and the limbic part of the striatum can influence the motor and association cortices.

The cross influence between closed circuits goes further than the level of striato-cortical connections. There are reciprocal connections between the striatum and the SNc, by which the dopaminergic input to the striatum is realized. There are closed and open components for the connections between each striatal area and its own dopamine (DA) system as well. Each striatal area reciprocally connects to a distinct DA area. This is the closed loop. However, each striatal area projects not only to a corresponding DA area, but also to other DA areas. For example, the motor part of the striatum projects not only to the motor

DA area but also to the limbic and associative DA areas, which project back to the limbic striatum and the associative striatum respectively. These are open loops affecting other striatum-DA system-striatum circuits.

Another open component in the circuits of the basal ganglia is related to the indirect pathways. An indirect pathway starts from the striatum, projects to GPe and to STN, and finally joins the direct pathway in GPi. However, there are projections from GPe to the functionally corresponding STN and also to functionally noncorresponding STN. For example, the associative GPe projects not only to the associative STN and then to the associative GPi, but also to the motor and limbic parts of the STN, and finally to the motor and limbic GPi. These are called *open indirect* routes (Joel & Weiner, 1998).

EVIDENCE OF THE BASAL GANGLIA'S INVOLVEMENT IN LANGUAGE

So far the structure of the BG has been described with the assumption that this structure is involved in procedural learning of a language. There have been many suggestions that the basal ganglia may subserve not only motor functions but also language functions (Aglioti, Beltramello, Girardi, & Fabbro, 1996; Blumstein, Alexander, Ryalls, Katz, & Dworetzky, 1987; Damasio & Damasio, 1992; Fabbro, 1999; Gurd, Bessell, Bladon, & Bamford, 1988; Klein, Zatorre, Milner, Meyer, & Evans, 1994, 1995; Lawrence, Sahakian, & Robbins, 1998; Lieberman, 2000; Lieberman et al., 1992; Ulman, 2001b; Ulman et al., 1997). This section presents evidence for the BG's involvement in language functions from three sources: animal experiments, disease studies, and lesion studies.

Animal Experiments

Laboratory animals undergoing motor sequence learning display characteristics similar to the ones that second language learners show as their proficiency improves. Jog and colleagues (Jog, Kubota, Connolly, Hillegaart, & Graybiel, 1999) inserted tetrodes in the striatum of rats that were undergoing t-maze training, a procedural learning task involving automatization. They found that the neuronal changes in the striatum and the changes in the rats' behavior correlate. The encoding of action in the striatum underwent dynamic reorganization as learning proceeded.

The rats had to run a t-shaped maze to reach a reward. They started running at the beginning of a T-maze when they heard an auditory signal. When they reached a point before the divergent t-shape, they heard another auditory signal. Depending on the sound, they had to decide whether to turn right or left. The rats received a reward if they reached the correct final point. With repetitive training, the rats' behavior improved in three ways. First, the reaction times to the auditory signal decreased, both for the initiation of the action and for turning direction. Second, the movement time from the starting point to the goal also decreased. Finally, performance accuracy increased. These behavioral changes are not unlike those of second language learners as they achieve greater proficiency.

Second language learners' linguistic behavior undergoes dramatic changes as their fluency improves. First, they initiate utterances more easily. This is parallel to the rats' ability to react faster to the signal for the initiation of action. Second, their reaction time in conversational turn taking decreases. When there are many native speakers and a second language learner in a conversational setting, it is difficult for the second language learner to take turns at the right moment. However, this becomes easier as his or her proficiency develops. This behavioral change is similar to that of rats when they learn to react faster to the signal for turning. Third, with increased fluency, second language learners can comprehend and produce utterances of the target language faster. This change is similar to that of the rats when the total movement time to reach the goal decreases. Finally, the learners obtain greater accuracy in their use of the target language in a way that parallels the rats' increased performance accuracy. This analogy does not prove that the motor learning in the rats and SLA are the same process, but it is sufficient to show that they have much in common.

Second language learners experience tremendous difficulties until they acquire a certain degree of fluency. I speculate that the difficulties are caused because the second language learners have not had enough opportunities to automatize their second language through the BG. Therefore, with more opportunity for practice and increasing procedural memory of their target language though the BG, automatization will proceed, and greater fluency will be achieved.

Huntington's Disease, Parkinson's Disease, and Obsessive Compulsive Disorder (OCD)

Huntington's disease is caused by the degeneration of striatal medium spiny neurons that project to the GPe. Due to this degeneration, the indirect pathway becomes nonfunctional, and the direct pathway becomes abnormally efficient in disinhibiting the thalamus. This results in abnormal excitation of the cortex.

The resulting behavior is hyperkinesias, such as ballistic and choreic movements, which are the over-execution of motor routines (Purves, 1997; Ullman et al., 1997; Ullman, 2001b).

The abnormal behavior of Huntington's disease patients goes beyond hyper motor activity; these patients have abnormal linguistic behavior, as well. Ullman and his colleagues (1997, 2001b) have shown that the patients over-regularize irregular verbs and that they multiply suffixed forms. For example, they may change the verb to an incorrect past tense form (e.g., "dig" to "dugged", instead of "dug"; "look" to "lookeded", instead of "looked"). Their error rates correlate with the severity of their hyperkinesias. The bottom line is that the degeneration of the medium spiny neurons of the striatum causes overapplication of rules in language as well as in motor activity. Moreover, the pathology is consistent with what can be expected from IP malfunction.

Parkinson's disease also demonstrates involvement of the BG in language functions. Parkinson's disease stems from the loss of dopaminergic neurons in the SNc, which project to the striatum, amplifying cortical signals that activate the DP. Due to the lack of input from the SNc, the activation of the DP is weakened. Therefore, the ability to execute motor activity, or more generally, to execute routines, is compromised. Carlson summarized their symptoms as a "failure of automated memories" (Carlson, 2001, p. 454). The characteristics of Parkinson's disease patients are generally called *hypokinesia*, or paucity of movement (Parent, 1996; Purves, 1997).

Parkinson's patients also show impairments in linguistic behavior. Ullman and his colleagues studied these patients and identified their linguistic problems (Ullman et al., 1997; Ullman, 2001b). The patients' speech samples are grammatically very simple, with few or no compound sentences. They show deficits in both regular and irregular verbs, but their performance with irregular verbs is much better than with regular verbs. This distinction is relevant for understanding the role of the BG in language. For example, in languages such as English, regular verbs need the application of rules in order to be conjugated; irregular verbs do not. Distinct past tense forms may be remembered separately, and thus, declarative memory will suffice. As previously discussed, the direct pathway of the BG is needed to execute motor and cognitive routines and to apply rules. The fact that Parkinson's patients show deficits in conjugating regular verbs is consistent with what we can expect from the weakened or malfunctioning DP.

Obsessive compulsive disorder (OCD) also indicates that the BG is involved in linguistic function. This disease is caused by abnormal metabolic activity in the caudate nucleus of the striatum as well as in brain structures such as the orbito-frontal cortex and the anterior cingulate. These areas participate in the associative split circuit, which is the normal feedback loop that determines not only which sequences should be chunked, but also which sequences should be executed depending on the circumstances. Due to disruption of this loop, OCD patients cannot decide which chunk of motor or cognitive behavior is appropriate in a given situation. As a result, they repeatedly execute the same motor routines, and the same thoughts and ideas continuously emerge (Graybiel, 1998). OCD patients also display perseveration in linguistic behaviors. They tend to repeat the same words, phrases, or utterances impulsively. This repetitive linguistic behavior is what one could expect from malfunctioning associative split circuits, and clearly demonstrates that the BG is critically involved in language.

Lesion Studies: Aphasia

Aphasic syndromes caused by BG lesions indicate what roles the BG may play in language functions. According to Fabbro (1999), basal ganglia aphasics develop symptoms such as reduced voice volume, foreign accent syndrome, perseveration, and agrammatism. Additionally, a polyglot's more fluent language tends to be more seriously damaged than a less fluent language.

First, foreign accent syndrome is particularly relevant to this discussion. In the past, it has been thought to be simply disrupted motor control of oral articulatory organs. However, a few studies have questioned this interpretation. According to Klein et al. (1994), foreign accent syndrome is "a symptom clearly distinct from dysarthrias or apraxias of speech (p. 2296)." This argument is consistent with those of others (Blumstein et al., 1987; Gurd et al., 1988; Volkmann, Hefter, & Lange, 1992). Foreign accent syndrome is very likely to be caused by disrupted procedural memory—that is, the loss of the ability to execute phonological rules, which govern the realization of phonemes according to their environment. Children may acquire the phonological rules of their native language implicitly through procedural memory, and execute the rules automatically. It is not surprising that a lesion in the BG results in the disruption of phonology because the BG is responsible for rule formation and application.

Second, another symptom of patients with basal ganglia lesions is perseveration (Fabbro, 1999). Perseveration is "the involuntary repetition of syllables, words, or syntagms" (p. 40). This linguistic behavior is reminiscent of OCD, which is caused by pathological metabolism of the BG, especially the caudate nucleus. Although Fabbro did not indicate the exact location of the BG lesion, it may include the caudate nucleus, because the patients with lesions in this area frequently display repetitive and intrusive over-execution of motor or cognitive routines, including over execution of some verbal routines.

Third, agrammatism is generally observed in BG aphasics. They show disruption of grammar, and they especially tend to omit grammatical morphemes. Linguistically speaking, grammatical bound morphemes lack semantic content. They only show the grammatical relationship among constituents of sentences. For example, when one says "he goes", "he" and "go" have semantic content but "-es" after the end of the verb "go" does not. The morpheme "-es" may be processed by our unconscious knowledge of grammar rules. Therefore, when the neural substrates subserving rules are damaged, the parts of sentences having semantic content ("he" and "go") will be processed by other parts of the brain related to semantics, but other components of the sentences lacking in semantic content (e.g., the third person singular morpheme –s) may not have such a recourse. The fact that the patients with BG lesions omit grammatical morphemes indicates that the BG is involved in language functions, especially in grammar rules.

Finally, polyglots with lesions in the BG present a particularly interesting pathology to those who study SLA. When a polyglot suffers a basal ganglia lesion, all of the languages he or she speaks tend to be damaged. However, they exhibit a strange symptom called *paradoxical aphasia*, in which a second or foreign language tends to be less impaired than the patient's mother tongue. Aglioti and his coworkers (1996) reported such a case. Their patient (E.M.) suffered a basal-ganglia lesion, mainly in the neostriatum. After the insult, she exhibited Broca's aphasia, including agrammatism, in both her first language (Venetian) and second language (standard Italian). However, her first language was more affected than the second language. Contrary to the normal pattern for bilinguals, she also had greater difficulty in translating her second language into her mother tongue than vice versa. Similar instances were also observed by Fabbro and Asher (1999), Fabbro and Paradis (1995a, b), Aglioti and Fabbro (1993), and Fabbro (1999). Although the pathology of paradoxical aphasia may appear counterintuitive, this paradoxical situation is exactly what one would expect from a patient with a BG lesion.

The interesting fact that the patients' second languages are better preserved may imply that their second languages are processed more by the declarative memory system (see chaps. 4 and 5 of this book) than their first languages are. Although the automatization of a second language through the BG is ongoing, it may not be complete. When a patient suffers a BG lesion, the parts of the second language that have already been proceduralized will be damaged, but other parts of SL that have not been proceduralized will be preserved. In contrast, a first language may have been almost completely proceduralized without leaving much of a trace in the declarative system. This may be why BG-lesion patients cannot produce their first language in spite of their intact declarative memory system. This may also be why the second language of a BG-lesion patient is relatively better preserved.

THE BASAL GANGLIA AND SECOND LANGUAGE ACQUISITION RESEARCH

Knowledge about the BG functions may have important implications for the area of linguistics in general and SLA in particular. This section presents some research agendas for SLA that arise from our knowledge of the BG and procedural memory.

Learning Fixed Expressions: Chunking

Some researchers have noticed that second language learners tend to learn frequently co-occurring words as delexicalized chunks (Sinclair, 1991; Tannen, 1989). This phenomenon may be explained by the chunking mechanism of the BG. Previously, we discussed how the BG participates in the process of chunking the cortically distributed information into a unitary sequence through convergence, divergence, and reconvergence. The implication of this phenomenon for SLA may be related to our learning of fixed routine expressions of the target language such as idioms (*by and large*), ritualized expressions such as greetings (*glad to meet you.*), and other fixed expressions or collocations. Whenever a second language speaker uses one of the fixed expressions, he or she may simply activate the relevant basal ganglia circuit so that he or she does not need to apply a grammar rule or a phonological rule step by step.

Automatization of Syntax and Phonology: DP and IP

Learning and producing the phonology and grammar of a target language probably involve both the direct pathway and the indirect pathway. Through numerous and repetitive inputs of the target language and its production, a second language speaker may slowly build up stronger synapses among participating neurons in the cortex and basal ganglia, which represent the syntactic and phonological rules of the target language. Finally the learner acquires the ability to execute the rules through the direct pathway of the BG .

For example, the choice of word order may be the result of basal ganglia function. Whenever a second language speaker utters a sentence, perhaps there may be two competing word orders in the speaker's brain, one probably from his or her first language and another from the target language. When the speaker gets into the target language mode, the target language order may be executed through the direct pathway with the competing order being inhibited by the indirect pathway.

Other aspects of grammar may be the same. For example, an ESL learner is repetitively exposed to sentences in the present tense that have a subject in the third person singular and the verb that agrees with the subject in terms of number (Mary *looks* pretty today rather than *Mary *look* pretty today). With repetitive exposure to and production of such sentences, the learner is likely to slowly acquire the ability to execute the correct number agreement rule through the direct pathway and suppress the other possible verb forms through the indirect pathway.

Phonology is likely to develop in the same way. For example, in American English, the voiceless alveolar stop [t] is pronounced as a flap [ ] between a vowel and an unstressed vowel as in *water* and *matter* (Celce-Murcia, Brinton, & Goodwin, 1996). The rule could be 'whenever there is a sequence of vowel, voiceless alveolar stop, and unstressed vowel, the voiceless alveolar stop is pronounced as a flap.' As the learner improves his or her fluency in the target language through numerous repetitions in listening and speaking, he or she may acquire the ability to execute this rule through the direct pathway, and the pronunciation of /t/ as [Q] will be executed in that environment and the pronunciation of /t/ as [t] may be inhibited through the indirect pathway.

Formation of Rules of the Target Language

The formation of correct rules is often a difficult process. To form a correct rule, a speaker has to frequently execute the correct sentences related to the rule. However, a beginner cannot execute the correct sentence easily, and every time he or she executes an incorrect sentence, the wrong rule will be strengthened in the relevant neuronal circuits. A paradoxical situation is unavoidable here. The more often a beginning speaker utters incorrect sentences, the stronger the neuronal circuits representing them may become. However, advanced second language speakers conform to the rules of the target language to a greater extent than beginners. The question is how a second language speaker may avoid forming an incorrect rule? The answer may be found in the fact that the formation of rules is also affected by factors other than pure repetitive execution and exposure to the target language. I present here two possible factors: modulation by the dopaminergic system and intervention by declarative memory.

As previously explained, the BG includes two dopaminergic systems. First, the SNc, which contains dopaminergic neurons, projects to the striatum to amplify cortical signals and to facilitate the direct pathway. Second, the limbic closed circuit, which also includes dopaminergic inputs, comprises one of the five closed circuits of the BG. This circuit also affects other circuits through the open components of the BG. Schumann (1997, 2001a, b) showed how the neurotransmitter dopamine could affect the behavior of a second language learner. The dopaminergic system is pivotal for the appraisal and motivation that drives a learner to seek to improve or to give up (Matsumoto, Hanakawa, Maki, Kimura, & Graybiel, 1999; see also chap. 2, this volume). If the execution of a sentence, or a rule, is successful in conveying what a second language speaker wants to express, the cortico-basal ganglia neurons that represent the rule may form stronger connections through dopamine facilitation. If the execution of a sequence or a rule fails to get the desired result, the sequence or rule may not form stronger connections because dopamine facilitation will not take place. In the case of a beginning learner, if the interlocutor does not understand, the learner will be motivated to try a reformulation.

In addition to successful communication, many other factors may affect the dopaminergic system in a second language situation. A positive or negative response from the listener or a teacher can be one. A second language speaker's interlocutor may give feedback by a positive response such as "your English is good" or a negative response such as misunderstanding or error correction. If the speaker gets a positive response, the execution of the utterance may generate dopamine facilitation, and the utterance may form a stronger circuit (i.e., the beginning learner gets praise for using a correct utterance, and then the use of that construction will be reinforced). A negative response may generate the opposite result.

Intervention by declarative memory (see chaps. 4 and 5) may be another factor that influences the formation of the rules through the BG system. As previously discussed the limbic closed circuit of the BG originates from the hippocampal complex and entorhinal cortex. These systems are involved in declarative memory. This circuit can influence other circuits through the open components of the BG. Second language speakers, especially those receiving instruction, are likely to form declarative memories for the grammatical and phonological rules of the target language. For example, an ESL learner is likely to have learned and stored in his or her declarative memory system that the number of the subject and the verb must agree. When he or she utters a sentence that violates the rule, his or her declarative memory may send a signal indicating that the utterance is wrong. This signal may prevent the formation of connections among neurons that could have represented the incorrect rule. On the other hand, when the speaker executes a correct sentence, this information aligns with that of declarative memory, and the connection that represents the sentence or the rule involved in the sentence may become stronger.

Learning versus Acquisition

The previous section provides information that may help address an important issue that has been hotly debated in SLA. Krashen (1977, 1985) argued that there are two independent knowledge systems in a second language speaker: the acquired system and the learned system. The first is formed through innate language learning abilities, or a mental language organ, and constitutes the subconscious memory for grammar of the target language. It functions automatically. In contrast, the learned system is built via formal instruction, and involves conscious knowledge for the grammar rules. According to Krashen, these two systems operate independently, thus knowledge from one system cannot cross-over to the other. This claim, which was motivated by Chomskian UG theory, was interpreted to have implications for classroom language instruction. Krashen argued that because fluency in the target language is acquired—not through formal instruction, but through innate language learning abilities of humans—what language teachers have to do in classrooms is only to provide the students with comprehensible input. This theory gave birth to a teaching methodology called the *communicative approach*, which is still widely accepted and practiced in language classrooms all over the world today.

However, neuroanatomy provides an interface between learning and acquisition when learning is viewed as declarative knowledge and acquisition is viewed as procedural knowledge. This anatomy allows declarative memory to influence the development of procedural memory. As shown in Fig. 3.4, the declarative memory system and the procedural memory system share the same cortical areas. The cortical areas are likely to affect declarative memory (learning) and procedural memory (acquisition). Moreover, the hippocampus, which participates in declarative memory, is connected with the basal ganglia, which participates in procedural memory, and they influence each other. Our

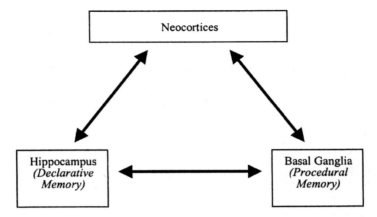

FIG. 3.4. Schematic representation of the interrelationship between declarative memory and procedural memory.

hypothesis is that the same neural system that allows declarative information to become procedural also operates to repair procedures that are inaccurately acquired and perhaps fossilized.

Fossilization and Defossilization

Fossilization has been a prominent topic among SLA researchers (Harley & Swain, 1978; Selinker & Selinker, 1972). We may be able to explain this phenomenon better by using information about how the BG works. Wu (2000) proposed that, as second language proficiency advances, the target language knowledge becomes "a set of regularized subroutines for planning and producing TL utterances" (p. vii). During the process, "(1) signals generated during planning and production are concatenated into coherent sequences; (2) learned sequences are consolidated into holistic units; and (3) holistic units are mapped onto neural representations of the context in which they typically occur" (p. vii). This process of routinization is thought to result in fossilization. For Wu, fossilization is critical evidence that this automatization is involved in the process of second language learning.

Wu argued that fossilized second language patterns are formed through years of repetition; they are resistant to alteration or suppression; they function independently of executive control, and are cognitively impenetrable. These characteristics of fossilized second language structures conform to the characteristics of automatization that are mediated by the basal ganglia. Wu, revising the model of Levelt (1989), proposed a three-step language production model. According to the model, the speaker must: (1) identify a goal and conceptualize a message, (2) construct utterances, and (3) prepare for articulation. In this process, step 1 is more under executive control than step 2, which, in turn, is more under executive control than step 3. On the other hand, step 3 is executed more automatically than step 2, which, in turn, is more automatic than step 1. Because of the characteristics of each step, fossilization appears most strongly at the phonological level, which mostly involves step 3.

Fossilized language speakers have two important characteristics (Harley & Swain, 1978; Selinker & Selinker, 1972). One is that they have already acquired a certain level of communicative fluidity. They can generate utterances in the target language without undue cognitive planning and without consciously building structures. They show less hesitation when engaged in conversation. In summary, their speech has fluency. Another characteristic of fossilized second language speakers is that their learning has stopped or radically slowed down. Their typical utterance structures and phonology do not improve over time although they may be continuously exposed to the target language environment. They continue to make the same grammatical and phonological errors although they are sometimes aware that they are doing so.

These two characteristics may be explained by BG functions and procedural memory. The first characteristic of fossilized second language speakers, natural fluidity, occurs because they have already acquired the target language procedurally, thus, they have obtained automaticity. By repetitive use of the target language, the speakers may have formed procedural memory of (incorrect) linguistic rules of the target language through the basal ganglia circuits. When one acquires a procedural memory of a motor or a cognitive skill, one can execute it automatically. This may be why some fossilized second language speakers can speak in the target language with automaticity.

The other characteristic of the speakers, rigidity of errors, can also be explained with reference to the BG and procedural memory. As discussed in the introduction of this book and previously in this chapter, procedural memory is formed more slowly than declarative memory. The other side of the coin is that procedural memory is more robust so that, once formed, it is better preserved, and it is also inflexible, and therefore difficult to change. This is why it is so difficult to correct bad habits in playing sports or musical instruments. If a fossilized second language speaker has already automatized the linguistic skills through basal ganglia circuits, the automatized skills are naturally resistant to correction and change. From these observations, we may be able to define fossilization as what occurs when some aspects of a second language have been proceduralized through the basal ganglia but these elements do not perfectly conform to the rules of the target language.

An outstanding question is whether fossilized language can be defossilized. Also, if it can be defossilized, what is the underlying neural mechanism? First, defossilization perhaps is possible. Although fossilized rules are resistant to alteration and suppression and cognitively difficult to penetrate, they are not impossible to change. It is not too rare to meet fossilized speakers in a language classroom. Some of them come there with the intension of making their language use conform more to that of the target language. Although it is difficult for them to change their ingrained linguistic habits, many of them improve at least in some aspects. This change may be possible for two neurobiological reasons. First, the brain is always plastic, although the extent of plasticity varies according to many factors. Because the brain maintains plasticity, it is not impossible to form a new rule or to correct an incorrect rule. Second, the anatomy of the brain shows that the procedural memory of the basal ganglia can be influenced by other components.

To convert declarative knowledge into procedural knowledge or to restructure an incorrectly learned procedure with declarative information involves getting signals from the hippocampal system into the basal ganglia system. In Fig. 3.5, we suggest the anatomy that may underlie these processes. The hippocampus, with declarative knowledge, and the amygdala, with motivational involvement, both project to the ventral (limbic) striatum. This area of the brain, as we saw in chapter 2, is important in reward and in the conversion of incentive motivation into motor action. The ventral striatum connects to the basal ganglia via projections to the globus pallidus, and via the ventral pallidum, and it also projects to the brainstem motor nuclei and the spinal cord. Both the ventral pallidum and the globus pallidus influence the motor cortex via the thalamus. Dopamine (DA), which is involved in motivational modulation of its targets, is very important in this system, projecting from the ventral tegmental area and the SNc to the amygdala, the ventral striatum, the ventral pallidum, and the dorsal striatum.

From experience, we all know that automatizing declarative knowledge or altering a habitual procedure is difficult and time-consuming. It requires practice and the motivation to sustain that practice. Animals probably acquire declarative and procedural knowledge together as they experience the world. With humans, the symbolic species capable of language, it becomes possible to

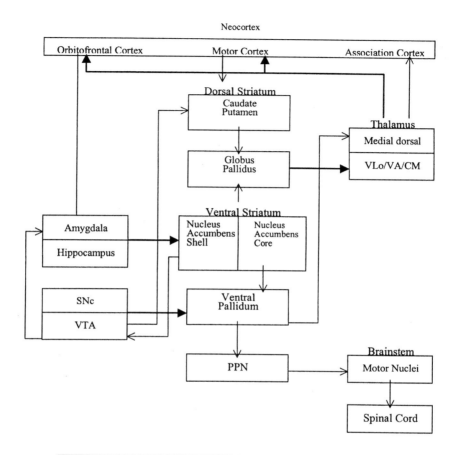

Neocortex

OFC-orbitofrontal cortex, SNc-substantia nigra pars compacta, VTA-ventral tegmental area, PPN-pedunculopontine nucleus, Vlo/VA/CM-motor thalamus

Declarative knowledge may become proceduralized and fossilization may become corrected via a system involving projections from the hippocampus and the amygdala to the ventral striatum, projection from the ventral striatum to the globus pallidus and the ventral pallidum, and dopamine innervation of the ventral and dorsal striatum.

FIG. 3.5. Diagram for fossilization and defossilization.

acquire declarative facts and procedural skill more separately. The split is particularly apparent in the acquisition of skill via declarative instruction, and classroom second language acquisition is a paradigm case of such learning. This type of learning requires cognitive work and the motivation to do that work. The task, of course, is facilitated by aptitude (see chap. 1).

From an evolutionary perspective, it is easy to understand why it may be difficult to alter motor procedures. Procedures are developed to help the organism thrive in the environment by allowing automatic responses to stimuli. If they were easily altered or disrupted, the animal's survival would be threatened. Therefore, when a language learner develops incorrect grammatical structure, these habit-protecting difficulties are encountered, and considerable effort is required to develop the correct procedures to override the maladaptive fossilization. As can be seen from Fig. 3.5, motivational input from the amygdala, the prefrontal cortex, nucleus accumbens, and the dopamine system is required to "power" the hippocampal declarative knowledge into the procedural system of the basal ganglia.

Declarative knowledge may become proceduralized and fossilization may become corrected via a system involving projections from the hippocampus and the amygdala to the ventral striatum, projection from the ventral striatum to the globus pallidus and the ventral pallidum, and dopamine innervation of the ventral and dorsal striatum.

CONCLUSION AND ADDITIONAL THOUGHTS ABOUT LANGUAGE

Second language learners utilize all types of memory to learn the target language. Lexical learning, semantics, and learning *about* the rules of the grammar and phonology of the target language probably involve declarative memory, which is based on the hippocampus and the neocortex (see chaps. 4 and 5, this volume). Learning grammar and phonology to the point of automatization may rely on the procedural system, which subserves motor and cognitive skills, and is based in the BG. As implied throughout this book, this chapter argues that learning a second or foreign language is achieved by domain-general learning mechanisms of the brain. Without presuming the existence of a specific module or any neural mechanism that subserves only language and nothing else, it is possible to describe the process of second or foreign language learning based on the anatomy and functioning of these general neural mechanisms.

Many issues in linguistics will be better understood by incorporating the information about the basal ganglia. This chapter discussed such linguistic phenomena as learning fixed expressions, learning morphosyntax and phonology, and fossilization and defossilization based on the mechanisms of the basal ganglia. However, this neural mechanism's implication for the linguistics does not stop here. Future studies may use the knowledge of this system to explore such linguistic issues as critical period phenomenon, transfer phenomenon, and diverse linguistic aptitudes among individuals, just to name a few.

4 The Neurobiology of Declarative Memory

Sheila E. Crowell

DEFINING LEARNING AND MEMORY

Introduction

The question as to how knowledge is acquired and stored has long been of interest to scholars and philosophers. Undoubtedly, all individuals have experienced the process of learning, remembering, and sometimes forgetting. Through these experiences humans have learned how to successfully navigate within their environment as well as how to alter that environment in ways that suit the survival of the species. In the past century, the study of learning and memory has become progressively more focused on the neural mechanisms at work in the brain. Now, with increasingly greater resolution, these studies are sufficiently detailed to allow researchers to make early hypotheses regarding the nature of human learning and memory storage.

Although it is difficult to biologically isolate the exact moment at which learning ends and memory begins, some scientists maintain the linguistic distinction between these two terms for explanatory purposes. One clear example of such a distinction is provided by Kandel, Schwartz, and Jessell (2000), who described learning as "the process by which we acquire knowledge about the world, while memory is the process by which that knowledge is encoded, stored, and later retrieved," (p. 1227). Yet whereas such definitions are useful, they are deceptively simple and possibly misleading in terms of the biological mechanisms that underlie these phenomena. First, in many instances it is not clear whether knowledge can be acquired without being simultaneously encoded at the cellular level. Second, the encoding, storage, and retrieval processes probably occur at multiple loci before the memory is finally stabilized in highly distributed networks in cortical regions of the brain (see chap. 5, this volume). Finally, this simple division between learning and memory implies a linear process from initial acquisition to final storage. However, it is more likely that memories that have been previously stored have already modified the brain in such a way as to affect the relative ease with which new memories can be formed. In other words, learning not only results in memory but is itself the result of memory. Therefore, at the cellular level, encoding, storage, and retrieval are represented as modifications in the strength of synaptic connections that are constantly being altered as the result of new interactions with our environment.

History of the Study of Learning and Memory

Although philosophers have long struggled with questions of how memories are stored, the beginnings of experimental research on learning and memory are frequently traced to the 1880s when German psychologist Hermann Ebbinghaus began to explore memory through objective and quantitative measures. Since that time, advances in chemistry and biology have increased the scientific desire to link behavioral experiments with what is known about the brain. Yet, due to the complexities of this organ, a growing number of scientists have realized that understanding learning and memory requires more than an analysis of brain functioning; theories regarding human behavior must also be developed. In the present chapter, this perspective is emphasized. Thus, connections between behavioral theories and observed biological processes are highlighted in an attempt to form accurate hypotheses regarding the nature of human mental function.

In the past 150 years, a number of important theories have been developed to explain the possible physiological mechanisms involved in learning and memory. One of the earliest of these theories, proposed by neuroanatomist Santiago Ramón y Cajal, is now considered to be the most plausible explanation of how memories are stored. Near the end of the nineteenth century a number of theories predominated. The first of these was that the neurons of the brain were not connected in a continuous chain but had a small gap between them; this small gap is now called the *synapse*. The second was that, once a nerve cell matures, it becomes limited in its ability to divide and multiply. Thus, it was believed that in a lifetime of experience, the number of nerve cells in the human brain might not increase significantly. These facts led Ramón y Cajal to suggest that the neuron might strengthen its connection with another neuron as a basic means of storing learned information. Although many scientists now believe that new nerve cells can be added to the brain—a process known as neurogenesis—the importance of synaptic plasticity as proposed by Ramón y Cajal is clear. In fact, "one of the insights of the modern biology of memory is the finding that the individual connection between two neurons is an elementary unit of memory storage," (Squire & Kandel, 1999, p. 29).

A more recent theoretical contribution to the field of learning and memory is that of Canadian psychologist Donald Hebb. Hebb's theory of learning can be summarized as follows:

When an axon of cell A is near enough to excite a cell B and repeatedly or persistently takes part in firing it, some growth process or metabolic change takes place in one or both cells such that A's efficiency, as one of the cells firing B, is increased. (Hebb, 1949 cited in Brown, Chapman, Kairiss, & Keenan, 1988, p. 725)

Hebb's Postulate suggested that when two neurons fire at the same time, a change will occur that will strengthen the connection between them. Historically, this property has been emphasized in the science of learning and memory because it shares the fundamental property of classical conditioning, "associativity" (Bliss & Collingridge, 1993). In other words, similar to the carefully timed pairing that must occur if the conditioned stimulus (CS) and the unconditioned stimulus (US) are to become associated with one another, there must also be a carefully timed pairing of activity at the presynaptic and postsynaptic neuron for them to become connected. Although Hebb developed his theory without concrete biological evidence, such neuronal associativity has now been observed throughout the brain and is believed to play a fundamental role in learning and memory. In fact, the type of associativity that Hebb predicted is so prevalent in the brain that synapses with these associative properties have been given the name Hebb, or Hebbian synapses (Martinez, Barea-Rodriguez, & Derrik, 1998).

Declarative Memory, Nondeclarative Memory, Consolidation, and Attention

The properties of Hebbian synapses were first described by Bliss and Lømo (1973), who provided a detailed account of the cellular processes involved in consolidation at the molecular level. This chapter begins to explain the importance of this early stage of consolidation in declarative learning and memory and the role that this form of consolidation may play in adult second language learning. Specifically, it explores how synapses come to be associated with one another in the Hebbian sense. However, this microlevel analysis is only able to provide a portion of the story; a detailed reading of the other sections of this book is essential for a number of reasons, the most important of these being the dynamic nature of the brain itself. In particular, it is essential that readers of this chapter follow by reading chapter 5, which is a further elaboration of the neural mechanisms involved in declarative memory.

Consolidation at the molecular level, which is the primary focus of this chapter, is the first stage of a long process of memory storage. This stage includes the strengthening of the connection between two neurons, and assumes that these two neurons are part of a constellation that is activated by a given set of stimuli. The constellation, or web of activation that is firing in response to a learning situation, may become associated in a neural network. In the pages that follow, a detailed description of the early stages of consolidation are given in relation to declarative memory. For the sake of simplicity, the term *molecular consolidation* is used to differentiate the consolidation that takes place at the molecular level (as discussed in this chapter) with "trace-transfer consolidation" (discussed in chap. 5). These terms are drawn from Nader, Schafe, and LeDoux (2000b). As we show in this chapter and the following, declarative memories are originally processed by—and eventually stored in—those cortical areas of the brain that are initially activated by a given set of stimuli. In the case of linguistic input, there is a strong tendency for the frontal and temporal cortices of the left hemisphere to be involved in decoding this type of information. However, just as with all types of information, the storage of linguistic stimuli requires a network of structures in the brain that extends far beyond the cortical areas in which the stimuli are eventually stored. In the case of adult language learning, for example, proceduralized linguistic input may eventually be stored in the neocortex, but only after making a loop through the circuits of the basal ganglia (chap. 3). This chapter introduces yet another subcortical structure, one that all declarative memories must loop through before they are stored in the cortex. The process by which memories are transferred from subcortical areas to the cortex is also known as consolidation or, more specifically, as *trace-transfer consolidation* (see chap. 5). It is important to understand that the molecular consolidation discussed in this chapter is not only the first stage of memory storage, it also underlies the transfer of information from the cortex to the subcortical areas involved in procedural and declarative memory, as well as the transfer from those subcortical areas back to the cortex. In other words, the relay of all information in the brain is rooted in the strengthening and weakening of connections between pairs of individual neurons. The following pages introduce the considerable literature on how neurons strengthen their connections and the role that this may play in the formation of declarative memories.

THE BIOLOGY OF DECLARATIVE LEARNING AND MEMORY

Locating Memory in the Brain

By the middle of the 20th century, there was a wide body of research localizing various mental functions in specific areas of the brain. A significant portion of that research was done by Wilder Penfield (Penfield & Rasmussen, 1950), who stimulated various areas of the brain in epileptic patients undergoing surgery. The vivid memories experienced by a small number of Penfield's patients after temporal lobe stimulation led him to suggest that some aspects of memory might be located in the temporal lobes of the brain. Although most scientists believe that memory storage involves various regions of the brain, it is clear that some areas are more important than others in the formation of certain types of memories (Kandel et al., 2000). One structure in particular, the hippocampus, which is located bilaterally on the medial surface of the temporal lobes, is now believed to play a crucial role in the formation of new declarative memories.

The Role of the Hippocampus in Learning and Memory

The first direct evidence linking the hippocampus to learning and memory came in 1957 when Canadian psychologist Brenda Milner and neurosurgeon William Scoville first reported on the case of their patient H.M. In order to cure H.M. of his severe epileptic seizures, Scoville surgically removed the inner surface of H.M.'s temporal lobe bilaterally, including the hippocampus and surrounding structures in the medial temporal region. Although this procedure proved to be an adequate remedy for H.M.'s seizures, the removal of the hippocampus rendered H.M. unable to form new declarative memories. Furthermore, after his surgery, H.M. experienced retrograde amnesia and thus was unable to remember those events occurring in the years prior to his operation, although his memory for more distant life events remained intact. This fact has led many researchers to suggest that the hippocampus be considered a temporary store for long-term memory, with more permanent storage of episodic and semantic knowledge occurring those association areas of the cerebral cortex that originally processed the information (Kandel et al., 2000). Yet exactly how "temporary" a role the hippocampus might have in memory storage is still a matter of debate. Recent research (Nadel, Samsonovich, Ryan, & Moscovitch, 2000) indicates that the hippocampus may play a role in the consolidation of certain types of memory for an indefinite amount of time. Specifically, Nadel, et al. (2000) proposed that although semantic knowledge may eventually become stored in cortical networks that are independent of the hippocampus, episodic knowledge may remain permanently linked to hippocampal traces (see chap. 5 for a more complete review of this debate).

Another crucial aspect of H.M.'s impairment was the fact that it was not accompanied by any deterioration in personality, general intelligence or in the ability to perform complex perceptual tasks. Reviewing this interesting spectrum of deficits and abilities, Scoville and Milner came to the conclusion that "the anterior hippocampus and hippocampal gyrus, either separately or together, are critically concerned in the retention of current experience," (Scoville & Milner, 1957, p. 11). Since that time it has become clear that the hippocampal region and the numerous pathways connecting that region to cortical areas are vitally implicated in the formation of new declarative memories as well as the eventual consolidation of those memories in cortical regions of the brain.

Location and Structure of the Hippocampal Region

The hippocampal region consists of a group of brain structures located deep inside the medial temporal lobe. These structures include the hippocampus, dentate gyrus, subiculum, and entorhinal cortex (Gluck & Meyers, 1998). Within this region information flows into and through the hippocampus via three major pathways:

1. The perforant pathway, which connects the entorhinal cortex to the granule cells of the dentate gyrus.
2. The mossy fiber pathway, which connects the granule cells of the dentate gyrus to the pyramidal cells of the cornu ammonis (CA) 3 region in the hippocampus.
3. The Schaffer collateral pathway, which connects the CA3 region of the hippocampus to the CA1 region (Squire & Kandel, 1999).

In a model proposed by Kandel et al. (2000), these unidirectional pathways, as well as other input and output pathways of the hippocampal formation, each play a specific role in hippocampus-mediated learning and memory formation. Information is first processed in the unimodal and polymodal association areas that are involved in the synthesis of sensory information, such as the frontal, temporal, and parietal lobes. Then, from these areas, information is relayed to the parahippocampal and perirhinal cortices, and then to the entorhinal cortex. Kandel et al. (2000) emphasized the dual role of the entorhinal cortex; not only does it send information from the cortex to the dentate gyrus, the subiculum, and CA3 and CA1 of the hippocampal formation, it also receives information from the hippocampal formation and relays that information back to the cortex. The input and output pathways that have been discussed to this point are depicted in Fig. 4.1.

The connectivity of the entorhinal cortex to both hippocampal and cortical structures make it critical in the consolidation of hippocampus-dependent memories. The consolidation process, which is discussed in more detail later, appears to entail multiple stages (see chap. 5 for the part of the consolidation process that includes the relay of information from the hippocampus to the cortex). The present chapter addresses one of the early stages of molecular consolidation, which involves the modification of neuronal ensembles in the hippocampo-entorhinal cortex system (Chrobak, Lorincz, & Buzsaki, 2000).

THE NEURAL BASIS OF LEARNING AND MEMORY

Long-Term Potentiation

As was first suggested by Ramón y Cajal, long-lasting changes in the strength or efficacy of synaptic transmission appear represent a cellular mechanism for the

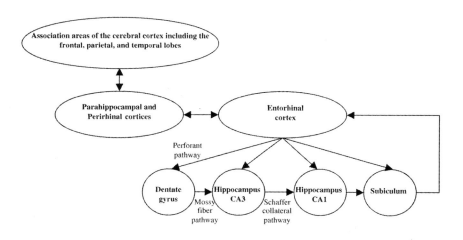

FIG. 4.1. Selected input and output pathways of the hippocampal formation.

storage of memories. Although some researchers still question the exact relationship between synaptic modification and learning and memory (McEachern & Shaw, 1996; Shors & Matzel, 1997), there is a large body of evidence linking changes in synaptic strength to how synapses function, both during development and during the storage of new information in learning (O'Dell, 1999). Currently, research on the cellular correlate of learning and memory has focused on two major phenomena, *long-term depression* (LTD) and *long-term potentiation* (LTP). LTD is characterized by a decrease in the efficacy of synaptic transmission, whereas LTP is characterized by an increase in the efficacy of synaptic transmission; the increase in synaptic connectivity resulting from LTP has been shown to last for days and even weeks. Although little is known regarding the exact role that individual neurons play in complex neuronal networks, a recent study looking at the activity of human hippocampal neurons proposes that both increases and decreases from baseline neural firing may be crucial to memory formation (Cameron, Yashar, Wilson, & Fried, 2001).

Since the discovery of LTP by (Bliss & Lømo, 1973), long-lasting potentiation and depression have been observed throughout the brain. Nevertheless, much of what is known regarding activity-dependent changes in synaptic strength comes from studies of the hippocampus, which may be because of the relatively simple anatomy of the structure as well as its suspected role in the formation of declarative memories (O'Dell, 1999). Furthermore, studies in the hippocampus have not always extended to all known types of hippocampal LTP, but have focused primarily on associative, N-methyl-D-aspartate (NMDA) receptor dependent LTP in the Schaffer collateral pathway. Because much of the core knowledge on LTP has grown out of this body of research, the primary focus of this chapter is to review what is known about associative LTP in the Schaffer collateral pathway. This is not to say that other forms of LTP, such as opioid-receptor-dependent LTP, which is found in the mossy-fiber CA3, lateral-perforant-path dentate gyrus, and lateral-perforant path CA3, are not important. It is clear that determining the role of the hippocampus in learning and memory will involve further research on the relationship between NMDA-receptor-dependant LTP and opioid-receptor dependent LTP (Martinez et al., 1998). However, unless explicitly stated, LTP is used in this chapter to refer to the type of potentiation that lasts for at least an hour and occurs in the Schaffer collateral pathway, which is associative and NMDA-receptor-dependent.

Properties of Hippocampal Long-Term Potentiation

There are a number of features of hippocampal LTP that make it critical to the study of learning and memory. In the hippocampus, LTP has been shown to occur in all three of the pathways through which information flows—the perforant pathway, the mossy fiber pathway, and the Schaffer collateral pathway (Squire & Kandel, 1999). The synaptic enhancement that occurs as a result of LTP is *rapid*, meaning the change can be induced by brief stimulation of an afferent input and *persistent*, meaning it lasts longer than other previously discovered types of synaptic enhancement (Brown et al., 1988). Furthermore, three basic properties of LTP "cooperativity, associativity and input-specificity," (Bliss & Collingridge, 1993, p. 31) appear to parallel some of the basic properties of learning and memory. Each of these features are discussed in turn.

Cooperativity refers to the specific strength and timing of neural stimulation that is required for the successful induction of LTP. In the laboratory, LTP is most conveniently induced by delivering a series of strong shocks, called a tetanus, to presynaptic neurons in the pathway that is being studied. A tetanus typically consists of a sequence of 50 through 100 stimuli that are administered at 100 Hz or more (Bliss & Collingridge, 1993). Two more moderate protocols that have also been successful are theta-burst stimulation, which consists of 4 shocks at 100 Hz each that are separated by 200 ms, and primed-burst stimulation, which typically involves a priming stimulus followed by sequence of 4 shocks at 100 Hz (Bliss & Collingridge, 1993). These specific patterns of shocks have probably been successful in inducing LTP because they mimic the high-frequency volleys that have frequently been observed in natural interactions between the hippocampus and the entorhinal cortex. Specifically, two distinct high-frequency volleys, *gamma/theta* (40-100 Hz) and *ripple* (140-200 Hz) have been observed in the entorhinal cortex and are believed to contribute to the natural formation of memories (Chrobak et al., 2000). In the neuron, cooperativity specifically refers to the fact that multiple afferent fibers need to be stimulated cooperatively. In other words, weak tetani that only activate a few afferent fibers will fail to induce LTP.

Associativity refers to the fact that both a presynaptic and a postsynaptic event are necessary for the enhancement of synaptic connectivity. Thus, as Hebb predicted, when two neurons fire at the same time one would expect to see a strengthening in the connection such that later, when one of those neurons fires, there is an increased chance that it will cause the other neuron to fire. This has been shown to occur in associative LTP, where the paired firing of the presynaptic neuron and the depolarization of the postsynaptic neuron lead to an enhancement of synaptic strength. In the early literature, associativity was often referred to as the cellular analogue of classical conditioning because even a weak (i.e., conditioned stimulus) stimulation to the presynaptic neuron, when paired with a strong (i.e., unconditioned stimulus) depolarization of the postsynaptic neuron can be sufficient to potentiate the cell (Bliss & Collingridge, 1993). This was considered to represent a possible physiological mechanism for encoding an association between two stimuli that are involved in firing the same group of target neurons (Geinisman, 2000). It is important to note, however, that the belief held by most researchers currently is that associative LTP is not the same thing as classical conditioning (Martinez et al., 1998). In other words, although classical conditioning may involve the potentiation and or depotentiation of a network of neural connections, it is impossible to say that any two neurons of the brain directly encode the relationship between two associated stimuli.

The final feature of LTP that makes it of interest in the study of learning and memory is *input-specificity*. Input-specificity refers to the fact that only afferents that have been stimulated show potentiation. In other words, LTP is homosynaptic, occurring only at the synapses where there has been a strong tetanus to the presynaptic cell. Yet recent studies have questioned the input-specificity of tetanized neurons, claiming that LTP induction might actually affect neighboring neurons. This, however, is not considered to be problematic since some flexibility may prove advantageous as compared to a strict Hebbian rule (Martinez et al., 1998).

Mechanisms of Long-Term Potentiation in the Schaffer Collateral Pathway

The Schaffer collateral pathway is the area of the hippocampus that connects the CA3 region to the CA1 region. Because LTP in this pathway is associative, it has been widely studied as a potential cellular correlate of Hebbian-type learning. Thus, the mechanisms of LTP in this area are well defined. Typically, LTP in the Shaffer collateral pathway has been studied in the brains of laboratory animals. In many of these studies, LTP has been artificially induced by an implanted stimulating electrode, which gives a tetanic stimulation to the presynaptic neuron. After this high-frequency stimulation, a number of changes occur that are critical in the long-term enhancement of synaptic connectivity. In the early literature on LTP, these changes were divided into three stages: induction, maintenance, and expression. Brown et al. (1988) defined induction as "the initial sequence of events that triggers or sets into motion the modification process," maintenance as "the factors that govern the duration of the enhancement," and expression as "the set of mechanisms that constitute the proximal cause of the synaptic enhancement," (p. 725). It is important to isolate LTP into these three different stages because of the increasing evidence from pharmacological studies (Malinow, Schulman, & Tsien, 1989) indicating that certain chemicals, when applied to the potentiated neurons, interfere with only one of these phases. Furthermore, if LTP is involved in learning and memory, then the induction phase should be associated with the initial storage of experience, the maintenance phase should correspond to the processes involved in converting that experience into a long-lasting memory, and the expression phase should be involved in the structural changes necessary for the permanent storage of the memory at the cellular level. As of yet, however, no direct link has been made between these three phases of LTP and distinct phases in memory formation.

Another important note regarding these phases of LTP is that scientists have recently begun to make less of a distinction between the maintenance and expression phases. This shift appears to be the result of the work by Eric Kandel, who typically divides LTP into an early phase and a late phase (Bailey & Kandel, 1993; Kandel et al., 2000; Squire & Kandel, 1999). In order to adequately address the wide body of LTP research, this chapter first describes the three phases that were initially considered important in LTP research—induction, maintenance, and expression—and then shows how these three phases map onto the newer descriptions made by Kandel.

LTP Induction

The induction of LTP in the Schaffer collateral pathway requires the cooperative activity of both the presynaptic and the postsynaptic neuron. In the presynaptic neuron, tetanic stimulation leads to the increased release of the transmitter glutamate. Glutamate binds with two types of receptors in the postsynaptic neuron, N-methyl-D-aspartate (NMDA-type) receptors and non-NMDA-type receptors. However, in typical synaptic transmission (without high-frequency firing of the presynaptic neuron), glutamate only activates the non-NMDA receptor, allowing for the influx of sodium (Na^+) ions into the postsynaptic cell—the NMDA receptor remains inactive because it is blocked by magnesium (Mg^{2+}) ions. Only with repeated stimulations to the presynaptic neuron is enough glutamate released to activate the NMDA receptor. In the NMDA receptor, we see the type of molecular association that was originally predicted by Hebb. This is because NMDA activation only occurs when two conditions are met: the glutamate released from the presynaptic neuron must bind to the postsynaptic receptor, and it must bind when there is a sufficient depolarization of the postsynaptic membrane. If both these conditions occur, the Mg^{2+} is expelled; the NMDA-receptor-gated channel opens; and both sodium

Na$^+$ and calcium Ca^{2+} enter the postsynaptic cell. Thus, much like the paring of the CS and the US, the successful induction of LTP requires presynaptic activity coincident with strong postsynaptic depolarization (O'Dell, 1999). Because NMDA-receptors are responsive to both the presynaptic release of transmitter and the postsynaptic depolarization, they act as "Hebbian coincidence detectors," and are thus responsible for the temporal and spatial summation that is viewed to be a fundamental property of associative LTP (Martinez et al., 1998, p. 218).

Although much of the literature on the mechanisms of LTP induction has been obtained through the process of artificially stimulating the presynaptic neuron, most scientists believe that similar high-frequency bursts of activity could occur naturally during the learning process (Squire & Kandel, 1999). Recent research (Brown, Frank, Tang, Quirk, & Wilson, 1998; Louie & Wilson, 2001; Siapas & Wilson, 1998) has provided electrophysiological evidence of patterned neural firing in the hippocampus of awake and moving rats. The ripple frequency volleys recorded during the learning of spatial tasks appear to be important for both the initial encoding of a task as well as its eventual consolidation as a memory. It is believed that this synchronized firing of ensembles of hippocampal neurons may, in fact, represent the ideal mechanism for the Hebbian modification of synapses (Louie & Wilson, 2001).

LTP Maintenance

Once the NMDA-receptor gated channels open, the influx of calcium into the postsynaptic cell activates a number of protein kinases. These kinases are considered important because they are believed to play a role in converting the induction signal (entry of Ca^{2+}) into a long-lasting change in synaptic strength (Bliss & Collingridge, 1993). Of these, the calcium calmodulin-dependent kinase (CaM kinase II) is believed to be particularly significant. First, CaM kinase II has been shown to enhance the ability of non-NMDA receptors to respond to glutamate, as well as contributing to the insertion of new AMPA (non-NMDA-type) receptors (Squire & Kandel, 1999). Second, CaM kinase II triggers a phosphorylation process in the postsynaptic neuron and, because "CaM kinase II activity is regulated by autophosphorylation ... [it] remains active long after Ca^{2+} levels have returned to basal levels," (O'Dell, 1999, p. 487). The ability of CaM kinase II to remain active for an extended period of time is what makes it possible for "long-term synaptic plasticity ... [to] last for years [although] all the molecules in our bodies, except DNA, turn over within days or weeks," (Kuno, 1995, p. 95). Third, CaM kinase II along with other protein kinases (such as proteine-cAMP dependent protein kinase—PKA) is believed to activate the enzyme NO synthase which acts on amino acid *l*-arginine to produce the gas nitric oxide (NO). NO diffuses out of the postsynaptic cell, moves back across the synaptic cleft, and into the presynaptic cell. It is now believed that NO is one of several substances that may serve as retrograde messengers; if the retrograde messenger reaches the presynaptic neuron while that neuron is firing, it will enhance the probability of continued transmitter release (Squire & Kandel, 1999).

The discovery that LTP maintenance might involve a chemical messenger that could travel from the postsynaptic neuron to the presynaptic neuron caused great interest in the scientific community. At the time, all previously discovered forms of chemical synaptic communication, other than gap junctions, were unidirectional—with messengers traveling from presynaptic terminals to postsynaptic receptors. Clearly, however, there are great advantages to this newly discovered form of synaptic communication. For example, let us suppose that normal (pre-LTP) synaptic communication involves a weak firing of the presynaptic neuron, which causes the release of one or two vesicles of the transmitter glutamate by the presynaptic neuron. If there is a strong input to the postsynaptic neuron, then there is a depolarization of the postsynaptic membrane from its normal resting potential (≈ -70mV) to ≈ -40 mV; the Mg^{2+} plug is expelled and the small amount of glutamate previously released by the presynaptic neuron is now sufficient to open the NMDA-receptor and allow for an influx of calcium. This pairing of a strong postsynaptic input (stimulating multiple afferent fibers) with a weak presynaptic input (stimulating only a few afferent fibers) is now sufficient to activate the chain of reactions leading to the production of the retrograde messenger NO. When NO reaches the weakly firing presynaptic neuron, it provides a strong signal for it to increase its firing and release more glutamate. In this way, a strong stimulus, if paired with even a weak stimulus, can lead to the enhanced connectivity of two neurons.[1] In essence, the retrograde messenger allows for the occurrence of long-lasting potentiation when sufficient amounts of postsynaptic depolarization occur in conjunction with presynaptic firing (Baranyi, Szente, & Woody, 1991).

LTP Expression

LTP expression, or late-phase LTP (Squire & Kandel, 1999) is the stage at which temporary short-term memories first begin the process of changing to more stable long-term memories. This process, known as consolidation, prob-

---

[1]This discussion of the associative pairing between weak and strong inputs is drawn largely from (Brown et al., 1988).

ably occurs at multiple levels before the memory can be considered "permanent," beginning in the hippocampus, with intermediate storage in hippocampo-entorhinal networks, and final storage in the cortical areas that were initially involved in perceiving the stimulus. At this point, we look at the consolidation that is occurring at the molecular level; further aspects of consolidation are discussed in subsequent chapters (see chap. 5 for a review).

LTP expression is characterized by a measurable increase in postsynaptic conductance (Brown et al., 1988), possibly resulting from structural changes such as "the addition into the presynaptic terminals of new release sites and the insertion of new receptors into the dendritic spines of the postsynaptic cell" (Squire & Kandel, 1999, p. 149). Structural changes in the postsynaptic neuron occur through a process of gene transcription. This process begins when repeated instances of LTP induction and maintenance heighten the amount of Ca^{2+} in the postsynaptic neuron to a level sufficient to activate the adenylyl cyclase enzyme. Adenylyl cyclase is important because it transforms adenosine triphosphate (ATP) into cyclic adenosine monophosphate (cAMP), a messenger that sends a signal to the cell's nucleus notifying it to begin expressing genes. The activation of the gene transcription process begins when cAMP interacts with protein kinase A (PKA), a by-product of the phosphorylation process. cAMP removes two regulatory subunits from the PKA structure such that it is able to diffuse into the cell nucleus. Then, PKA recruits the activity of the mitogen-activated protein (MAP) kinase, a kinase involved in cell growth. Together, these two kinases translocate to the nucleus, activating a genetic switch that causes the phosphorylation of transcription factors such as the CAAT-box enhancer-binding protein (C/EBP) and the cAMP-response element binding protein-1 (CREB-1). CREB-1 activates targets that are both regulators and effectors of growth, leading to the insertion of new postsynaptic receptors. C/EBP initiates the growth of new synaptic connections (Kandel et al., 2000; Squire & Kandel, 1999).

Figure 4.2 summarizes the mechanisms of LTP. The boxes on the left side of the diagram represent the activities occurring at the presynaptic neuron whereas those on the right represent the activities of the postsynaptic neuron. One starting point in this diagram is at the presynaptic neuron, where an increase in transmitter release leads to the depolarization of the postsynaptic neuron.

For a simple reading of the diagram, start at the presynaptic neuron on the left side at the top of the diagram. A high-frequency tetanus to this neuron causes it to release glutamate, which binds to receptors on postsynaptic neuron causing a depolarization—a reduction in the resting potential of the postsynaptic neuron. This depolarization forces the magnesium plug out of the NMDA receptor, which allows calcium to enter the postsynaptic cell. The

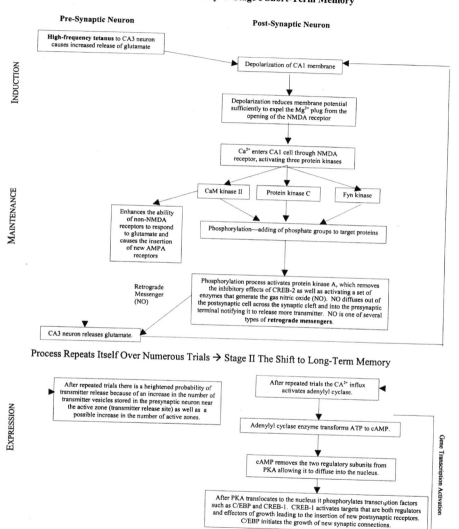

LTP in the Schaffer Collateral Pathway → Stage I Short-Term Memory

Pre-Synaptic Neuron   Post-Synaptic Neuron

INDUCTION

High-frequency tetanus to CA3 neuron causes increased release of glutamate

Depolarization of CA1 membrane

Depolarization reduces membrane potential sufficiently to expel the Mg^{2+} plug from the opening of the NMDA receptor

Ca^{2+} enters CA1 cell through NMDA receptor, activating three protein kinases

MAINTENANCE

CaM kinase II   Protein kinase C   Fyn kinase

Enhances the ability of non-NMDA receptors to respond to glutamate and causes the insertion of new AMPA receptors

Phosphorylation—adding of phosphate groups to target proteins

Retrograde Messenger (NO)

Phosphorylation process activates protein kinase A, which removes the inhibitory effects of CREB-2 as well as activating a set of enzymes that generate the gas nitric oxide (NO). NO diffuses out of the postsynaptic cell across the synaptic cleft and into the presynaptic terminal notifying it to release more transmitter. NO is one of several types of **retrograde messengers**.

CA3 neuron releases glutamate.

Process Repeats Itself Over Numerous Trials → Stage II The Shift to Long-Term Memory

EXPRESSION

After repeated trials there is a heightened probability of transmitter release because of an increase in the number of transmitter vesicles stored in the presynaptic neuron near the active zone (transmitter release site) as well as a possible increase in the number of active zones.

After repeated trials the CA^{2+} influx activates adenylyl cyclase.

Adenylyl cyclase enzyme transforms ATP to cAMP.

cAMP removes the two regulatory subunits from PKA allowing it to diffuse into the nucleus.

After PKA translocates to the nucleus it phosphorylates transcription factors such as C/EBP and CREB-1. CREB-1 activates targets that are both regulators and effectors of growth leading to the insertion of new postsynaptic receptors. C/EBP initiates the growth of new synaptic connections.

Gene Transcription Activation

FIG. 4.2. Mechanisms of LTP in the Schaffer collateral pathway.

entrance of calcium into the postsynaptic neuron causes a cascade of changes that eventually contribute to the generation of the retrograde messenger. The retrograde messenger signals the presynaptic neuron to release more glutamate, which then causes the process to continue (this begins with the release of glutamate from the presynaptic cell and leads to the depolarization of the postsynaptic cell—follow the arrow back to top). After this process occurs several times, the initial stages of molecular consolidation begin (see the second page of the diagram). Stage II, or late LTP, represents the shift to long-term memory and starts when CA^{2+} activates adenylyl cyclase. This initiates the gene transcription process that is necessary for consolidation to occur at the molecular level.

Structural Changes Resulting from LTP

Although it has been argued that LTP may result in synaptic remodeling and even in synaptogenesis, the research regarding the nature of post-LTP structural change is conflicting (Geinisman, 2000). At present, there is a general consensus that late-phase LTP involves some synaptic remodeling, such as the growth of additional presynaptic sites for the release of neurotransmitters and the insertion of new receptors into the postsynaptic membrane (Kandel et al., 2000). However, the notion that LTP may result in structural changes to the synapse is still highly contested. Some are adamant in their claim that no there is long-lasting change in the total number of dendritic spines in mature neurons post-LTP (Sorra & Harris, 2000), whereas others assert that LTP induction may have a significant effect on synaptic morphology, including an increase in the density of certain subtypes of synapses (Geinisman, 2000). Geinisman also claimed that the appearance of new spines is "significantly correlated with the degree of synaptic enhancement," (p. 959) indicating a strong relationship between LTP and synaptic growth.

The contradictory reports on the nature of post-LTP structural changes probably result from methodological differences between studies. Specifically, the increased number of synaptic contacts reported in Geinisman (2000) was shown to apply only to the number of perforated axospinous synapses in the dentate gyrus. Axospinous synapses are noteworthy because they are characterized by varying morphologies; some show a complete partition, with transmitter release zones on either side of the division, whereas others show no partition. Electron micrographs indicate the existence of various stages between zero and total perforation. Geinisman claimed that these morphological stages indicate phases in synaptic development from a less efficient synapse, with one transmission zone, to a more efficient synapse, with multiple transmission zones. Later, these axospinous synapses, with an increased number of completely partitioned transmission zones, may become an entirely different subtype of synapse, with entirely new connections. Accordingly, this may occur when the axospinous synapses convert into axodendritic synapses during a later stage of LTP (Geinisman, 2000). The hypothesis that axospinous synapses may convert into axodendritic synapses is based on the observation of a special subtype of perforated synapse that looks as though it might represent a transitional state between the axospinous-type synapse and the axodendritic-type.

The development of new perforated axospinous synapses is especially provoking if one accepts that this conversion is indicative of the well-researched scenario in which synapses that were previously silent become active. Long-term potentiation is believed to play an essential role in this conversion through the insertion of new alpha-amino-3-hydroxy-5-methylisoxazole-4- proprionic acid (AMPA) receptors into the postsynaptic membrane. AMPA receptors, which are part of the non-NMDA subtype of receptors, are crucial to normal synaptic transmission because, unlike NMDA receptors, they are not blocked by magnesium ions. Thus, they are of extreme importance in synaptic communication, where the stimulation is not strong enough to displace the magnesium block. Recent studies have shown that silent synapses can become active after LTP and have shown a causal relationship between LTP and glycine-facilitated AMPA receptor insertion (Lu, Man, Ju, Trimble, & Wang, 2001). Geinisman (2000) proposed that the reported increase in the ratio of perforated to nonperforated synapses may actually represent the morphological stages in the conversion of silent synapses to active ones.

Evidence Linking LTP to Learning and Memory

Although LTP is considered to be the primary model for how learning and memory storage occur at the synaptic level, the evidence supporting this claim is still inconclusive and speculative. This is because there are multiple forms of LTP, and because the distributed nature of memory storage in the hippocampus makes it difficult to understand the role of one potentiated neuron in a complex neural network (Martinez et al., 1998). Moreover, neither the properties of LTP nor those of memory are fully understood. For example, can the duration of a memory be correlated with the duration of potentiation? To this day, little is known regarding exactly how long memories, or the increased connectivity resulting from LTP, can last (Gallistel, 1995), although the claim is that both can endure for an indefinite amount of time. Regardless of these uncertainties, researchers have continued to study LTP and its role in learning and memory. From their work a new body of evidence has emerged, providing further support for the role of long-term potentiation in the acquisition and storage of new information.

Gene Targeting Studies

Gene targeting is a technique that is used to derive mice with mutations that are specific to a single cloned gene. This is accomplished by injecting mutant cells into an embryo, which results in offspring that are chimeras—mice carrying the mutant gene. The chimeric mice are then mated to produce a mutant line of mice. A number of different formulas have been used in gene targeting studies. One of the most common formulas is to create "knockout" mice by selecting a single gene and essentially knocking it out by inserting a bacterial gene, such as the neomycin resistant (neo) gene, in its place (Silva & Giese, 1998). The neo gene serves as a placeholder during recombination and is later removed, resulting in a mouse that is lacking the targeted gene. Another formula used in gene targeting studies is the creation of "transgenic" mice. In these mice the transgenic gene, such as CaM Kinase II-Asp 286, is introduced into the brain. CaM Kinase II-Asp 286 (a substitution of a threonine for aspartate D at position 286 of the protein) is placed under the control of a special promoter, for example *tet-O*, which is normally found only in bacteria. Unlike the normal promoter, *tet-O* cannot turn on the gene by itself. Rather, it must be activated by a specific transcription regulator, such as *tetracycline transactivator* (tTA) (Kandel et al., 2000). To create mice that carry both the *tet-O* promoter and the tTA transcription regulator, two transgenic mice (one with CaM Kinase II-Asp 286 attached to *tet-O* and one with tTA) are mated. In the resulting offspring the tTA binds to the *tet-O* causing the activation of the mutated CaM Kinase II gene, a mutation that leads to the over production of CAM Kinase II, which can seriously interfere with LTP. The transcription factor tTA is important in this process because it allows for the external regulation of the mutated gene. This is accomplished by giving the mice doxycycline, a drug that binds to the transcription factor tTA. When doxycycline is administered, it changes the shape of tTA, causing it to detach from the promoter. The cell ceases to over express CaMKII and LTP returns to normal (Kandel et al., 2000). In essence, the researchers are capable of turning LTP on or off. This allows for predictions as to the exact role of long-term potentiation in the learning and storage of the skills needed for a specific task.

Numerous variations of transgenic and knockout mice (as well as other animals) have now been created, each with a different mutation targeted to interfere with a particular aspect of LTP. However, the real question is: *does interfering with LTP cause deficits in learning and memory?* At this point, all that can be said is that disrupting the mechanisms involved in LTP may disrupt the processes needed for memory formation (Silva & Giese, 1998). For example, the CaMKII mice showed a significant impairment in the hidden-platform water maze, a task known to rely on hippocampal-dependent learning. These same mice, in an electrophysiological analysis, showed a change in the range of tetanic frequencies at which hippocampal LTP and LTD take place. This indicates that one possible role of CaM Kinase II is to set the threshold for LTP and LTD in synapses. It also suggests that LTP and LTD represent two ends of a biochemical continuum and that in these mice the frequency curve for LTP and LTD had shifted more towards LTD (Silva & Giese, 1998). Thus, in these mutants there was an impairment in the ability to learn as well as an impairment in long-term potentiation, indicating a clear correlation between the behavioral results (reduced ability to perform on hippocampal-dependant learning tasks) and the physiological evidence (the functional shift from LTP to LTD).

HUMAN LEARNING AND MEMORY

The Hippocampus and Associated Structures: Distributed Memory Networks

Even with the rich body of data accumulated on hippocampal LTP, the exact role of this structure in the process of learning and memory remains unclear. In fact, some have used the very fact that LTP occurs in the hippocampus to argue against the position that LTP is involved in memory storage (Gallistel, 1995). This argument is based on evidence from patients such as H.M., which indicates that long-term memories are not stored in the hippocampus and surrounding cortex. However, this argument ignores the fact that molecular consolidation is not the final stage of memory storage. Instead, the hippocampus is probably implicated in the initial stages of memory formation, in which the depression or potentiation of hippocampal neurons is crucial to the storage of information in a neural network. For this reason, understanding hippocampal LTP requires that we address the possible role of neural circuits, and how altering the weights of individual neurons through learning experiences can leave an imprint that may later be involved in recreating that experience as a memory (Silva & Giese, 1998).

Connectivity of the Hippocampal Region

As previously discussed, one of the primary connections between the hippocampus and the rest of the brain is through the entorhinal cortex. For this reason, studying the properties of entorhinal cortical neurons as well as their anatomical connectivity may reveal what role this area of the brain plays in memory formation. A recent study on the physiological patterns of neuronal ensembles in the hippocampo-entorhinal cortex system provides a preliminary review of oscillations in the brain, and how these oscillations may serve as a natural mechanism for translating experience into memory (Chrobak et al., 2000). Chrobak, et al. note that the neurons of the entorhinal cortex are organized into two distinct high-frequency patterns: *gamma* (40-100 Hz) frequency volleys, and *ripple* (140-200 Hz) frequency volleys. The ripple frequency volleys are found in layers V and VI of the entorhinal cortex, whereas the gamma frequency volleys are found primarily in layers I-III. The entorhinal cortex is organized such that layers I-III are involved in receiving information from cortical areas and relaying that information to the hippocampus; layers V and VI receive information from the hippocampus and then relay that information to cortical areas.

In the model proposed by Chrobak, et al. (2000) neocortical inputs are conveyed to the hippocampus through gamma frequency volleys. Thus, when an animal moves through its environment, layer II and III entorhinal neurons relay signals to hippocampal areas such as the dentate gyrus, CA1, CA3, and the subiculum. At this stage it is proposed that ensembles of entorhinal neurons are involved in actively changing the strength of hippocampal circuits to encode a particular experience. The authors also suggested that layer II of the entorhinal cortex may serve as a "novelty detector." For example, when a rat is placed in a familiar environment no changes in synaptic weight are necessary, thus the hippocampus simply outputs the previously stored neuronal representation. However, should the rat be placed in a novel environment, the entorhinal cortex will be involved in modulating changes in the synaptic strength of hippocampal neurons. In this case, the internal representation/prediction is relayed from the hippocampus to layers V and VI in the entorhinal cortex. This prediction is then compared with the external representation coming from the neocortex to layers II and III. As the external stimuli continue to influence the internal hippocampal representation, the output from the hippocampus will change to reflect new predictions about the environment. This process continues even when the animal is at rest or asleep and can be observed through distinct patterns of gamma frequency volleys. The persistent interactions between deep layers V and VI and superficial layers I-III are believed to continue until the internal representation/ prediction matches the external input and is likely to support a process of off-line memory consolidation (Chrobak et al., 2000).

There is a considerable body of literature suggesting that oscillations in the hippocampal area of the brain may play a fundamental role in the consolidation of memories during sleep (Wilson & McNaughton, 1994). This belief is supported by evidence linking patterns of neuronal activity during the awake behavior of trained rats to similar patterns observed while the rats were asleep. The consolidation process, to be discussed in greater detail in chapter 5, is believed to occur gradually and in a number of steps:

1. Connections from the hippocampus to the entorhinal cortex must be strengthened, whereas interhippocampal connections weaken.
2. Then the connections from the entorhinal cortex to the sensory areas of the neocortex must be strengthened, whereas hippocampo-entorhinal connections weaken.
3. Finally, cortico-cortico connections must strengthen, whereas entorhino-cortical connections weaken.

This transfer of information, known as a *memory trace*, or *engram*, is still not fully understood and remains a matter of great debate. Although the traditional model, articulated by Squire (Squire, Knowlton, & Musen, 1993), suggests that consolidated memories are eventually stored in cortical circuits that are independent of the hippocampus, recent research (Nadel & Moscovitch, 1998; Nadel et al., 2000) indicates that episodic memories may maintain traces in the hippocampus for an indefinite period.

Implications for Second Language Acquisition

Neural Studies

For obvious reasons, the role of hippocampal neurons in human learning and memory has been difficult to determine. There is little doubt, however, of the existence of LTP and LTD in humans, because these forms of neuronal plasticity are ubiquitous in living organisms from the fruit fly (*drosophila*), to the marine snail (*aplysia*), to mammals, such as mice and even primates. Some studies on human hippocampal neurons do exist, however, and are of great interest in understanding the possible biological mechanisms at work in the processing of complex tasks. For example, in one recently published article, a group of researchers looked at the activity of human hippocampal neurons during the encoding and recall of word pairs (Cameron et al., 2001). Their subjects included 12 adult epilepsy patients who agreed to have intracranial, depth electrodes placed bilaterally in their medial temporal lobes—approximately six electrodes per side in the amygdala, hippocampus, and entorhinal cortex. The electrodes were placed in areas that had not been affected by the epileptic seizures.

Subjects were presented with 20 word pairs, 10 that were related (dinner-food) and 10 that were unrelated (light-camp). After a brief delay period, the subjects were cued with the first word of each pair and were asked to respond verbally with the other word in the pair. The same words were presented later in seven alternating encoding and retrieval blocks. The activity of hippocampal neurons during the *encoding* stage was most predictive of later recall success. Both increases (8/13 neurons) and decreases (5/13 neurons) from baseline played a role in later memory for pairs. Interestingly, the word pairs that caused the greatest response in neuronal firing rate (either positive or negative increases from baseline levels) were the pairs that were later forgotten; those pairs that caused a smaller response were the ones that were subsequently remembered. Also, 3 of the 5 neurons that showed a decrease in firing activity whereas encoding remembered pairs, showed an increase in firing activity while encoding pairs that were later forgotten. This suggests that a complex network of interconnected hippocampal and entorhinal neurons are activated by verbal learning tasks.

Although the authors do not hypothesize as to why larger responses[2] in firing activity correlated with forgetting, whereas smaller responses correlated with remembering, there are several possible explanations for these results. One could be that the neural firing did not actually reflect verbal encoding but rather subject expectations. For example, it may not be surprising for a subject to see a word pair such as dinner-food and therefore may not cause much activity at the neural level. Word pairs that were surprising to the subject may have caused greater activation but that activation may have had nothing to do with remembering. Instead, it would just mean that more unusual pairs were harder to remember. Another possibility is that encoding word pairs that are rarely associated requires more effort than encoding word pairs that are frequently associated. This would suggest that less neural activity is required for tasks that are simpler, a claim that is fairly controversial in the neurosciences.

---

[2]As indicated, responses refer to both increases and decreases from baseline activity.

In the study by Cameron et al. (2001) the activity of hippocampal neurons during the encoding stage of the task was predictive of later recall success. However, no such parallel was seen between the activity of the hippocampal neurons during the retrieval stage of the task and later recall success. Instead, the activity of *entorhinal* neurons during the retrieval stage seemed to show a pattern reflective of the successful recall of word pairs. In those entorhinal neurons whose responses could be correlated with accurate retrieval, an increase in firing rate was observed during the interval between the presented cue and the correct response. In short, Cameron et al. revealed a division of labor in the hippocampal formation, with the hippocampus involved primarily in encoding and the entorhinal cortex involved primarily in retrieval. Perhaps the true significance of this study is that it shows activity in the neurons of the hippocampal formation during a language related task. However, since the study only sampled a small number of neurons it is difficult to determine how neuronal increases and decreases contributed to the encoding and recall of the word pairs. It is most likely that each of these neurons represented only a single node in a complex neural network.

Imaging Studies

Because of the invasive nature of studies such as that conducted by Cameron, et al. (2001), imaging studies are clearly a more practical way to look at hippocampal activity in humans. Recently a number of studies using functional magnetic resonance imaging (fMRI) and positron emission tomography (PET) have begun to explore the involvement of the hippocampus and the surrounding areas in the medial temporal lobe (MTL) during language-related tasks. Although early studies failed to show MTL[3] activation during language tasks (e.g., Shallice et al., 1994), a number of recent studies have shown language related activity in this area (Dolan & Fletcher, 1999; Fernández, Brewer, Zhao, Glover, & Gabrieli, 1999; Fernández et al., 1998; Heun et al., 2000; Johnson, Saykin, Flashman, McAllister, & Sparling, 2001; Martin, 1999; Saykin et al., 1999; Wagner et al., 1998). However, it is important to note that "activity" in fMRI studies merely indicates that a particular area is involved in a task; fMRI technology is unable to indicate whether that activation is excitatory or inhibitory.

---

[3]In earlier imaging studies the hippocampus and the cortical areas surrounding it were often discussed as a part of the medial temporal lobe since the imaging protocols of those studies did not allow for more specific claims regarding the location of activation. More recent studies have imaged just the hippocampal formation and have provided more precise statements regarding hippocampal regions involved in various tasks.

There is considerable controversy within the neuroimaging literature regarding where in the hippocampal formation verbal encoding and retrieval occur. Recent research using PET and fMRI suggests that encoding leads to activation in anterior portions of the hippocampal formation (including the dentate gyrus, subiculum, and entorhinal cortex) whereas retrieval causes activation in posterior portions of the hippocampal formation (Lepage, Habib, & Tulving, 2000; Small et al., 2001). These findings contradict earlier work indicating that verbal encoding takes place in posterior regions (Fernández et al., 1998). Other studies have not mentioned an anterior/posterior distinction but have claimed that encoding of words involves only the entorhinal cortex (Fernández et al., 1999), the parahippocampal gyrus (Wagner et al., 1998), the left hippocampus more than the right (Martin, 1999), and even the right hippocampus more than the left (Johnson et al., 2001). Regardless of these conflicting data, all of the mentioned studies agree that the hippocampus is needed for some aspect of verbal learning and memory.

One of the earlier studies done by Wagner et al. (1998) showed that during a verbal encoding task, greater activation in the left medial temporal cortex was associated with words that were later remembered and less activation was seen in words that were forgotten. They also found that subjects had better memory for words that required semantic processing (looking at a word and determining if it is abstract or concrete) rather than nonsemantic processing (looking at a word and determining if it is printed in upper (or lower-case letters). This evidence supports the instincts of many language teachers—students simply learn better if they attach meaning to what they study.

Another study looking at verbal encoding and recall found that subjects with greater activation in the right hippocampus as compared to the left scored better on the California Verbal Learning Test (CVLT) (Johnson et al., 2001). The authors proposed that this may be because participants with greater memory capacity might be engaging more sophisticated encoding strategies, including the use of imagery or the formation of complex associations between words. Unfortunately, the authors did not report asking the subjects how they went about processing the information. Thus, the idea that the right hemisphere was activated as the result of imagery or the formation of associations is just a hypothesis.

Although the majority of these studies deal with the encoding and retrieval of lexical items, there is one study that looked at artificial grammar encoding (Dolan & Fletcher, 1999). This study is particularly important for understanding the neural basis of second language acquisition, as traditional linguistic theory would not expect hippocampal involvement in grammar learning; the hippocampus, after all, does not appear to be specifically involved in language or unique to the human brain. The experimental design of Dolan and Fletcher's experiment consisted of six separate encoding blocks. Within each block, the subjects viewed six presentations of ten different items—five of the items represented grammatical strings and five of the items represented ungrammatical strings. Subjects were asked to identify whether the string was or was not grammatical and were given immediate feedback regarding the accuracy of their response. With this experimental design, the researchers were able to look at both the explicit learning of specific strings (within-block analysis) as well as the gradual learning of the grammar system (across-block analysis).

As Dolan and Fletcher had anticipated, the within-block analysis revealed initial left anterior hippocampal activation that gradually decreased as the subjects became familiar with individual strings. This finding is consistent with the work discussed earlier, which has shown that encoding activates the anterior hippocampus. The across-block analysis showed a similar effect; in this case, the anterior MTL region also showed an initial increase in activation that declined with a greater understanding of grammatical rules, this decline was seen even if the exact string was entirely new. In other words, the decrease in activation really did reflect an increased familiarity with the grammaticality of strings. The posterior MTL region—the left parahippocampal gyrus to be precise—showed a gradual increase in activation as the learned rules were applied to new situations. In short, learning a rule system appears to follow basically the same pattern of activation as learning individual exemplars within the rule system. Based on these results one might conclude that adults learning a second language use the same system—namely the network of structures involved in declarative memory for learning both the lexicon and the grammatical rules of a second language.

Second Language Theory

In the literature on second language acquisition (SLA), there has been considerable debate as to whether second languages are acquired declaratively, nondeclaratively, or through some combination of the two processes. The research presented in this book (chaps. 3 and 5 in particular) should make it clear that both the declarative and the nondeclarative memory systems are necessary for language acquisition. In other words, the parallel activity and interconnectivity of the basal ganglia system with the hippocampal system make it clear that both nondeclarative and declarative learning will naturally take place in any language-learning scenario. However, it may be the case that immersion learning is slightly more procedural in nature, whereas classroom learning is slightly more declarative. Although in the past several decades, some teaching methods have endeavored to change this. Guided by Krashen's input hypothesis (Krashen, 1982), a number of teachers have attempted to teach second languages simply by providing comprehensible input that is one step ahead of the students level (I+1). This theory proposes that students do not need explicit instruction but can gain language skills implicitly, continually progressing one step at a time. According to Krashen, second language *acquisition* (a subconscious process) is different from and is not the result of second language *learning* (a conscious process) (Krashen, 1994). In other words, there is no interface between learning and acquisition.

The noninterface position held by Krashen may be better understood by looking at second language acquisition from a neurobiological perspective. Though Krashen himself did not attempt to make a biology-based argument, there are several possible biological assumptions inherent in his position. These are:

1. The areas of the brain involved in subconscious processes (acquisition) are different from those areas involved in conscious processes (learning). That is to say, declarative and nondeclarative learning are accomplished by different areas of the brain.
2. There are no connections between these two brain regions.
3. The declarative system cannot modulate activity in the nondeclarative system. In other words, practicing an explicitly learned rule over and over again will not help the learner to strengthen connections in areas of the brain responsible for proceduralization.

Currently, SLA theorists are moving away from Krashen's noninterface position, and are taking the stance that rule acquisition in language is a complex cognitive task that lies on the same power function learning curve as other cognitive skills (DeKeyser, 1997). These researchers suggested that SLA is similar to the acquisition of most skills, which appear to involve interactions between the declarative and the nondeclarative memory systems (Berry, 1994; Ellis, 2000; MacWhinney, 1997). Ellis, for example, discussed three likely ways in which implicit and explicit knowledge might interact in language learning. First, explicit knowledge might be converted into implicit knowledge if the learner is at the right stage of linguistic development. Second, explicit knowledge may lead the learner to listen for a recently learned language structure in the input. Third, explicit knowledge might cause learners to notice the difference between their own output and the output of native speakers (Ellis, 2000). These three points are not only borne out by observations of adult language learners, they are also true of the underlying biology. Perhaps only the first of the three points needs some revision based on the research presented in this book. Specifically, we would assert that knowledge that is stored declaratively is not *converted* into nondeclarative knowledge. Instead, learners acquire and store information in both declarative (hippocampus/cortex) loops and nondeclarative (basal ganglia/cortex) loops. Thus, what would appear on the behavioral level to be a "conversion" is, in actuality, probably a strengthening of connections in the nondeclarative loop that is *sometimes* accompanied by a weakening of connections in the declarative loop. I emphasize the word "sometimes" because of the research presented in the previous chapter noting that fluent (i.e., highly proceduralized) speakers of a second language are often able to recover their second language, presumably because that information is still represented in the declarative system of the brain (see chap. 3 for a more thorough review).

A recent article that has analyzed the interface between the two memory systems is MacWhinney's commentary on implicit and explicit processes in second language acquisition (MacWhinney, 1997). In this article, the author cited a number of sources claiming that second language learning is facilitated by explicit instruction. However, he also suggested that implicit learning may still play an important role in the acquisition of a second language. Further, MacWhinney suggested that explicit instruction may actually be harmful if the structures that are being taught are too complicated, irregular, or simplified to the point of being incorrect. To conclude, MacWhinney suggested that future studies should look at how implicit and explicit learning processes aid in the acquisition of certain target structures. He asserted that both implicit and explicit processes may contribute to learning and that "in the end, the attempt to attribute language learning to either implicit or explicit processes will inevitably have to be answered by a position that emphasizes the contribution of both …." (p. 279).

The view of language as a complex task similar to other types of learning is supported by the fact that adult second language learners achieve variable success in the target language. Interestingly, it may be possible to partially account for individual differences among adult learners based on the basic mechanisms of LTP in the hippocampus. Specifically, it appears that there is considerable individual variation in the genes responsible for activating the transcription factors CREB and C/EBP, which are on chromosome two and chromosome sixteen, respectively (Ridley, 2000). These transcription factors, described in the final box of Fig. 4.2, are crucial to the growth and insertion of (1) new postsynaptic receptors (CREB) and (2) new synaptic connections (C/EBP) during the late phase of LTP. Gene knockout studies have revealed that without CREB and C/EBP, organisms are incapable of converting short-term memories into long-term memories. Moreover, in organisms where the gene activating CREB is particularly active, memory is significantly improved (Silva, Smith, & Giese, 1997). However, it is important to note that numerous factors probably contribute to the differential success seen in adult SLA. These probably include the individual's appraisal of the language learning situation along the five dimensions discussed in Schumann (1997, and chap. 2 of this book): novelty, pleasantness, coping potential, goal/need significance, self and social image. Other nongenetic factors contributing to individual variation in SLA might include prior learning experiences or similarity of the L1 to the L2 (i.e., a Spaniard learning Italian might have an easier time than a Korean).

A Language Learning Scenario

Up to this point, this chapter has reviewed the areas of the brain involved in the initial stages of declarative learning and memory. Furthermore, it has proposed that the strengthening of neural connections and the mechanisms involved in that process (namely LTP and LTD) may be important to several aspects of adult second language learning. The notion that the hippocampal region is involved in memory formation is now well accepted in the fields of neurobiology and psychology; what is not clear is whether adult second language learning involves the same areas of the brain that are involved generally in learning. Linguists are divided on this issue and, because it has been difficult to find proof for either side, the debate will probably continue. The following scenario presents a parallel account of the learning of a grammatical rule and the biological mechanisms discussed in this paper.

If it is assumed that the student is sufficiently motivated and has chosen the language classroom as one way to achieve proficiency in a second language, we can begin to look at the learning mechanisms that the student might engage. In the classroom, the student receives visual, auditory, and sometimes tactile input—with most teachers presenting information in various modalities. At the earliest levels of language instruction, many teachers follow the format of the basic introductory text. These books are set up in a fairly uniform manner, first presenting a grammar rule, then providing some form of practice, rule then practice, rule then practice, and so on. As the student engages in these tasks, the neurons of the brain are firing. The cortical areas involved in the initial processing of these linguistic stimuli probably form a complex neural network; such areas might include frontal lobe regions, which are involved in working memory, attention, and the formulation and organization of linguistic utterances; temporal lobe regions, which could be activated if the student is listening to linguistic input or if the task triggers memories from the student's past; and finally, motor, sensory, visual, aUp to this point, this chapter has reviewed the areas of the brain involved in the initial stages of declarative learning and memory. Furthermore, it has proposed that the strengthening of neural connections and the mechanisms involved in that process (namely LTP and LTD) may be important to several aspects of adult second language learning. The notion that the hippocampal region is involved in memory formation is now well accepted in the fields of neurobiology and psychology; what is not clear is whether adult second language learning involves the same areas of the brain that are involved generally in learning. Linguists are divided on this issue and, because it has been difficult to find proof for either side, the debate will probably continue. The following scenario presents a parallel account of the learning of a grammatical rule and the biological mechanisms discussed in this paper.nd auditory cortices, which could all be engaged depending on the task requirements. This multimodal input is pulled together in the association areas of the cortex.

Studies on humans and on animals suggest that the information stored as explicit memory is first processed in one or more of the three polymodal association cortices (the prefrontal, limbic, and parieto-occipital-temporal cortices) that are involved in the synthesis of auditory, somatic, and visual information (Kandel et al., 2000). From these multimodal cortical areas, information is relayed to the parahippocampal and perirhinal cortices, to the entorhinal cortex, through the hippocampus proper, and then back to the cortex via the same pathway. In the hippocampal region, the earliest stage of memory formation most likely involves the firing of neuronal ensembles in layers I-III of the entorhinal cortex, which are the primary areas involved in relaying information from the cortex to the hippocampus proper (Chrobak et al., 2000). In the language learning process, for example, the hippocampal neurons would probably be initially activated during the encoding of the vocabulary items and grammatical rules that are presented in the textbook. This encoding process would occur as the student navigates through the text, comparing the newly presented words and rules to those with which he or she is already familiar.

From this point, the information travels through the hippocampus proper, where the new information induces changes in the hippocampal neural circuits. As a result, the information is delayed en rout to the cortex in layers V and VI of the entorhinal cortex, the layers responsible for relaying hippocampal input to the cortical areas of the brain (Chrobak, et al., 2000). Chrobak, et al. propose that layers V and VI are responsible for comparing the previously learned information, which is stored in hippocampo-entorhinal networks with the new information that is being encoded. This comparing process continues until the difference between the old representations and the new representations is resolved. In terms of language, the student would most likely be comparing one grammatical form or lexical item to other familiar forms or items that were recently studied. In such a case, the hippocampus would be activating some of the neurons involved in previously stored networks while simultaneously activating several new neurons. Chrobak et al. believe that the information cycles through the hippocampo-entorhinal network until there is no conflict between this previously stored knowledge and new information. It is through this process that a new neural network might be formed.

As the student becomes increasingly familiar with the rule (by reading it repeatedly and by completing exercises), the neural connections between the hippocampus and the entorhinal cortex may begin to weaken and connections between the association cortex and other cortical areas may begin to strengthen. After some time, this type of semantic linguistic information may become entirely independent of its hippocampal traces (see chapter 5 for some debate on this issue). At this point, the learning is complete and, as was the case for H.M., activating the memory no longer requires the hippocampus.

The following two figures are loose adaptations from the work of Chrobak et al. (2000). In order to clarify the previous discussion on the possible neurobiological mechanisms involved in the learning of lexical items and grammatical rules, it may be helpful to review this process step by step. To do this, let us consider two different scenarios; one in which the student is rehearsing a familiar grammar rule and one where the student is learning a new grammar rule. The starting point in Fig. 4.3, the familiar situation, is at the gray number one with the color gray representing the input.

For the purposes of discussing this familiar situation, it may be useful to consider a case where the adult student is practicing the simple present tense. In the simple present tense the student must build a sentence that follows the rule: *subject* + *base form of a verb* + *-s* (in the case of third person singular) + *predicate*. For example, the teacher might ask the student to describe a scenario that would involve the use of the simple present tense, such as describing what the character, Jane, does every day. The teacher's request triggers the activation of neurons in the association cortices of the brain, which is the first step of the process. To read the diagram, follow the gray (1) from the cortex to the parahippocampal and perirhinal cortices, then (2) to the entorhinal cortex, then (3) to the subiculum of the hippocampus, and then (4) back to layers V-VI of the entorhinal cortex. From the subiculum (4) the information makes one cycle from entorhinal deep layers V-VI to entorhinal superficial layers II-III. When the input reaches layer II of the entorhinal cortex, entorhinal neurons trigger

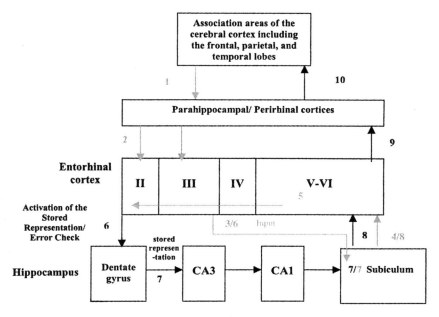

FIG. 4.3. Schematic depiction of the role of the hippocampal formation in the execution of a recently learned but familiar rule.

the activation of the stored representation that most accurately represents the input (most likely based partially on the information that layer II has received from the firing of subicular neurons that were triggered by the input stream). In the present scenario, the activation of the stored representation (black 6) will include the learned rule structure for constructing the simple present tense. Through the activation of the stored representation, layer II of the entorhinal cortex essentially serves as a novelty detector/error checker. Indeed, the primary function of neurons in layer II of the entorhinal cortex is to compare the neuronal representations from the neocortical (bottom-up) inputs with feedback (top-down) inputs from the hippocampus, essentially to resolve the discrepancy or "error" between the two (Chrobak et al., 2000). In a case such as the present one, where the input and the stored representation match, the hippocampus simply sends the familiar representation (6) to the subiculum, where both the firing patterns from the cortical input (gray 7) and the stored representation (black 7) are involved in activating layers V-VI of the entorhinal cortex (gray/black 8). Because the stored representation and input match there is no need for layers V-VI to reactivate layer II of the entorhinal cortex for further error correction. Thus, the familiar pattern can be sent to the cortex, allowing the student to correctly construct the rule for the simple present tense.

Figure 4.4 depicts a more complex scenario—one where the student must learn a new rule and therefore must reconstruct the stored representation.

In this second scenario, let us consider a situation where the student is learning how to put together a new sentence—only now in the present progressive tense. To form such a sentence the student would need the following rule: *subject + auxiliary be (conjugated) + base form of verb + -ing + predicate*. To encourage the student to form a sentence using the rule for the present progressive a teacher might ask the student to say what the character, Jane, is doing right now. Thus, in lieu of a familiar construction such as *Jane eats in the dorm cafeteria every day*, the student would now need to build a new sentence such as *Jane is eating in a restaurant right now*. There are obviously a number of similarities between these two sentences, which leads to the present hypothesis that the

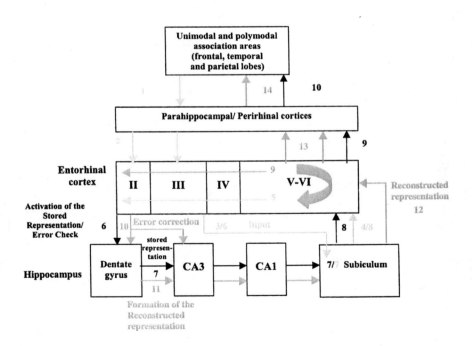

FIG. 4.4. Schematic depiction of the role of the hippocampal formation in the construction of a new neural network during the learning of a new rule.

learning of the present progressive tense would likely fire several populations of neurons that overlap with the rule for the simple present.

Similar to Fig. 4.3, follow the input (gray 1- 5) from the cortex, through the entorhinal cortex, to the hippocampus and then back to EC layer II. As before, layer II is responsible for firing the stored representation in the population of hippocampal neurons (black 6-8) and, also as before, the stored representation will represent a familiar rule such as that for the simple present tense. This time, however, a mismatch or error will be detected within layer II. This error triggers the process whereby a new neural network is formed, a process that begins when the conflicting information from the stored representation (black 8) and the input (gray 8) both send their conflicting output to EC layers V-VI. As a result of this conflict, EC layers V-VI do not send the stored representation back to the cortex as in Fig. 4.3, but rather continue sending the information to layer II for a comparison between the old and new representations (dark gray 9) and the formation of the reconstructed representation (dark gray 10,11,12) begins. This process continues until the mismatch is resolved (see the dark gray circular arrow representing an iterative process) and a new network, containing some neurons of the old representation and some of the new one,[4] is formed. When this process is completed the correct output will be generated and sent to the cortex (dark gray 12,13,14). One might hypothesize that, until the formation of the new representation is complete, the student might actually produce some blend of the old form and the target form. This is frequently observed in the language classroom when students say things such as *"Jane is go to the store every day,"* or *"Jane go to the restaurant right now."* This assertion would be a logical extension of the hypothetical language learning scenarios that have been presented in this section.

In the interpretation of this and the previous figure, it is important to understand that information in the brain does not travel from one end of an arrow to another. Instead, the interactions between the hippocampus and the entorhinal cortex probably occur as patterned firings of populations of neurons with information from the entorhinal cortex to the hippocampus being relayed at the theta/gamma frequency, whereas that from the hippocampus to the entorhinal cortex is firing at the ripple frequency (Chrobak et al., 2000). Clearly, interactions in the brain cannot be presented accurately in a linear figure, as there is no starting point and no ending point for neural activity; the brain is a dynamic organ that engages in parallel processes and, as a result, does not lend itself well to static illustrations.

---

[4]Note that the color dark gray was chosen to represent the overlap of the neurons that fire in response to the novel input (gray), with the neurons that fire in response to the stored representation (black).

It is likely that there are significant individual differences in the number of cycles through the hippocampus that are needed for each student to learn a rule, as well as differences in the number of cycles required for different rules for the same student. While some students may immediately recognize the discrepancy between the two forms and rapidly begin producing target-like utterances, other students may take weeks or even months to resolve this conflict. One reason for this difference is that each student's brain has been shaped by idiosyncratic experiences (see chap. 1). Furthermore, as was previously discussed, this difference between students may partially result from individual differences in the genes responsible for activating the transcription factors CREB and C/EBP. Thus, because the process of shaping the reconstructed representation involves the formation of new neural connections and the selective strengthening or weakening of other neural connections, those students who have a lower threshold for the induction of LTP may require fewer learning trials. This model, although still hypothetical, could account for numerous aspects of second language learning.

CONCLUSION: THE NEUROBIOLOGY OF SECOND LANGUAGE LEARNING

This chapter has offered a possible neurobiological account for the declarative learning of second language lexical items and grammar rules. The presented model analyzed the process of declarative learning on multiple levels, beginning with the microscopic interactions between two neurons, continuing with the formation of neural ensembles in hippocampo-entorhinal circuits, and concluding with the cognitive process of learning a second language. This formulation is based on a logical extension from research in the fields of neurobiology and psychology. However, until technology advances significantly, the hypothesis that adult second language learning involves the neural processes described in this chapter cannot be demonstrated. As such, we can only begin to get at this issue indirectly. For example, future research could include more neuroimaging studies on the encoding of foreign language grammar rules. Scientists working with individuals who have hippocampal lesions may want to look at what aspects of a second language can be learned when the hippocampus is damaged or missing. Finally, it would be interesting to continue the work that has been done in populations that have to undergo temporal lobe surgery for epilepsy. Wherever possible, researchers should continue to collect data from patients who have recording microelectrodes implanted in their hippocampi. This would allow for more accurate conclusions to be drawn about the nature of hippocampal involvement in higher cognitive functioning.

Although it is clear that there is still much to be discovered about the processes of learning and of forming memories, the research presented here reveals that learning and memory can now begin to be understood at the molecular level. The important work to be done will extend beyond the neuron to higher mental activity in human beings. With this goal in mind, this chapter represents the first attempt to build a theoretical model for how declarative learning may occur in the brains of adult second language learners. In essence, this work is representative of a relatively new scientific movement, one which begins with molecules and endeavors to explain the mind.

5   The Neurobiology of Memory Consolidation

Nancy E. Jones

One hotly debated topic in second language acquisition and studies of bilingualism has been the status of the "bilingual lexicon." Research into the neurobiological aspects of the "bilingual lexicon" has focused on studies of aphasics and psycholinguistic studies of normals. Recently, the role of declarative memory in lexical learning and storage has been emphasized (Paradis, 1994; Ullman et al., 1997), but none of these studies has determined a mechanism for lexical learning. If memory is an essential element for learning, then the biological mechanisms for memory should underlie lexical learning as well. Although this chapter focuses on the role of declarative memory in lexical learning, this mechanism should not be considered exclusively limited to lexical learning. It is an example of how a general cognitive mechanism can be seen as a mechanism for language.

To discuss the role of memory in language learning, we must first understand how the memory systems function. Within this framework, a number of concepts in memory formation are relevant to language learning. The first is how *newly* acquired knowledge is transformed from a new memory into a stable memory that can be accessed at a later time. This is the issue of memory consolidation. A corollary issue is how *old* information can be accessed and retrieved at a later date. This is the issue of memory retrieval. Both of these issues and how they relate to lexical learning are discussed.

In this chapter, I review the major neurobiological theories and two neuropsychological models: the Standard Theory (Mueller & Pilzecker, 1900) and the Multiple Trace Theory (Nadel & Moscovitch, 1997) that deal with memory consolidation. Based on evidence from neuropsychological studies and from studies within the modulatory framework, I support the proposal that Multiple Trace Theory (MTT) is a more accurate memory theory. I further argue that the MTT is more suitable as a mechanism for language learning. Specifically, I show how the MTT can adequately explain lexical learning. With an adequate model for lexical learning, there is no need to propose a "lexicon" in the brain—lexical items are not located in a generalized lexicon module, but rather are located in the regions involved in the processing of the semantic features of the word or to the type of input (auditory, visual, or motor).

DEFINITION OF CONSOLIDATION

The term *consolidation* has been used to describe the necessary changes to neurons (molecular changes) and more broadly to describe the development of neural systems for long-term memory. Nader, Schafe, and LeDoux (2000a) identified three major approaches to the study of consolidation. The first is the *molecular consolidation theory*, which focuses on the cellular and molecular events related to the development of long-term memory. Nadel and Moscovitch (1997) referred to these initial molecular changes as cohesion—a short-term consolidation process—which is the beginning of long-term consolidation. Fuster (1995) referred to this aspect of the process as the gateway to long-term memory. This first stage of consolidation is discussed in detail by Crowell (chap. 4, this volume). The second approach is *modulation-of-consolidation theory*, which focuses on how the strength of memory representations is affected by hormonal influences. Finally, the third approach is *trace-transfer consolidation theory*, which focuses on the transfer of memory over time between brain areas (specifically from the hippocampus to the neocortex; Nader, et al., 2000b). Neuropsychological theories can be characterized as *trace-transfer theories*.

Generally, during consolidation, there is a close and on-going relationship between the association areas in the neocortex and the hippocampus. As memories are formed, information comes into the hippocampus via the entorhinal cortex from the sensory and association areas in the cortex. Activity in the hippocampus is coordinated with activity in the neocortex. This is achieved by sending information back to the neocortical areas or by coordinated actions of the hippocampus and the cortical areas (Nader et al., 2000b). The trace-transfer theory is primarily concerned with these processes whereas much of the work in molecular and modulatory consolidation theory, focuses on molecular processes in the hippocampus when short-term memories are first being consolidated.

NEUROBIOLOGICAL APPROACHES TO CONSOLIDATION

Molecular Consolidation Theory: Cellular Processes of Consolidation

As discussed in chapter 4, studies in aplysia and rats show that the transformation of short-term memory to long-term memory requires the synthesis of new proteins (Bailey, Bartsch, & Kandel, 1996; Bailey & Kandel, 1993). These new proteins lead eventually to cell growth (Squire & Kandel, 2000). This process begins in the late phase of LTP, in which genes for "feedback regulators" are "switched on". Following this is the transcription of proteins necessary for the growth of new synaptic connections (Squire & Kandel, 2000). It is this structural change that distinguishes long-term memory from stable short-term memory (Squire & Kandel, 2000).

As just mentioned, memory consolidation not only requires hippocampal cellular changes, it also requires coordination of the hippocampus and the neocortical areas (McGaugh, 2000). Chrobak, Lorincz, and Buzsaki (2000) described the reciprocal pathways from the cortex and the hippocampus. The formation of a learned memory starts with information coming into the hippocampus from a cortical region involved in a particular type of learning task. Specifically, this information is received first by cell layers II and III of the entorhinal cortex and is then sent to the hippocampus where the molecular processes involved in the initial cellular consolidation of the memory occur (Chrobak et al., 2000). Consolidated information returns to the neocortical areas via cell layers V and VI of the entorhinal cortex (see also chap. 4). The cortical regions involved in memory formation vary according to the type of memory and type of input.

There are several cortico-hippocampal pathways, each associated with a specific type of memory. Take, as an example, the cortico-hippocampal pathways for a memory about an object in space, which includes both spatial and visual input. Rolls (2000) observed that in monkeys, both spatial information and visual information project to specific neurons in the hippocampus. These cells in the hippocampus make associations between spatial information (from the parietal cortex) and information about the object from other areas such as the inferior temporal cortex. According to these data, Rolls (2000) suggested that neurons in the hippocampus provide associative networks representing spatial position and neurons providing information about objects—associations that can be used to form memories about objects. The combination of this information culminates in the CA3 region. Information is sent back to the cortex from CA3 via CA1 and the entorhinal cortex. This information is then sent, via backprojections, to the areas of cerebral cortex that originally provided inputs.

There are also other cortico-hippocampal pathways for associative memories and semantic memories (Fuster, 1995; Squire & Kandel, 2000). For example, the frontal cortex is involved not only in working memory, but also in the consolidation of associative memories (Fuster, 1995). Laroche, Davis, and Jay

(2000) found that there is a direct monosynaptic connection between the ventral CA1 region of the hippocampus and prefrontal cortex. Semantic and verbal memories involve the inferior frontal cortex and the superior temporal cortex (Fuster, 1995).

Some of the areas in the cortex that have connections with the hippocampus are summarized in Table 5.1, which also shows the type of memory that is associated with the areas of cortex.

These cortical-hippocampal connections are important in understanding long-term consolidation.

Modulation Theories: Fear Conditioning and the Amygdala

The *amygdala*, a structure in the medial regions of the temporal lobe, plays two important roles in memory formation. It is crucial for the formation of fear-conditioned memories and is involved in modulating the intensity of all types of memories (McGaugh, 2000; Paré, Collins, & Pelletier, 2002). Modulatory substances in the limbic areas can make memories stronger or prevent consolidation of memories. They do this by interfering with the cellular processes necessary for consolidation. In his comprehensive review, McGaugh (2000) pointed out that the amygdala plays a key role in modulating memory consolidation. The amygdala is necessary for the formation of conditioned fear responses because the amygdala is the primary region involved in the regulation of emotion. It also modulates the consolidation of other types of memory through its β-adrenergic receptors. The β-adrenergic receptors in the basal lateral amygdala (BLA) are important for modulating the enhancing effects of glucocorticoids and hormones, which may come from other regions of the brain or body (Liang, Juler, & McGaugh, 1986 cited in McGaugh, 2000). McGaugh (2000) reported that amphetamine infused in the amygdala has been found to enhance spatial memory in rats. Ferry, Roozendaal, and McGaugh (2000) also found that stress-induced activation of the noradrenergic system modulates declarative memory storage.

TABLE 5.1
Cortical Areas Connected to the Hippocampus

Cortical area with a connection to the hippocampus	Type of memory
Parietal cortex	Spatial, tactile
Inferior temporal cortex	Visual
Superior temporal	Semantic

These studies demonstrate the amygdala's crucial role in memory modulation. The amygdala itself, however, is generally not considered to be a storage site for memories although there are some who believe that information is indeed stored in the amygdala (Fanselow & LeDoux, 1999).

NEUROPSYCHOLOGICAL APPROACHES TO CONSOLIDATION

As was stated in the introduction, neuropsychological theories emphasize the transfer of memory over time between brain regions and offer models of the brain systems involved in memory consolidation. Two neuropsychological theories of consolidation are the Standard Theory and the Multiple Trace Theory. The one theory that has dominated the study of the neural systems involved in memory consolidation is the Standard Consolidation Theory.

Standard Consolidation Theory

The standard theory of consolidation, first articulated by Mueller and Pilzecker (1900), characterized the development of long-lasting memory as a time dependent process. The formation of long-term declarative memories begins with a close relationship between the hippocampus and neocortical areas. Sensory information from the neocortex is processed by the hippocampus to create a trace or engram (McClelland, McNaughton, & O'Reilly, 1995; Squire, 1992; Squire & Zola-Morgan, 1991), which is formed by the molecular changes to the neurons in the hippocampus (Milner, 1999). It is likely that changes in the late stage of LTP constitute the formation of the trace (see chapter 4 of this volume for a detailed discussion of LTP). This is the beginning of the consolidation process. Through reciprocal connections, both the hippocampus and the neocortex are involved in the storage and retrieval of memories. Over time, the strength of the neocortical traces increases and the hippocampal connections are gradually weakened. Eventually, according to the Standard Theory, long-term memories can be stabilized in the neocortex and no longer depend on the hippocampus for storage and retrieval. This means that older memories, which are stabilized in the neocortex, would be less susceptible to disruption or damage in the hippocampus than newer memories.

This theory draws support largely from studies of amnesic patients (see Squire & Alvarez, 1995 for a review.) Evidence for this theory comes from Scoville and Milner's (1957) study of the case of H.M. (see also chap. 4). H.M. underwent bilateral removal of the hippocampus and adjacent structures. Although H.M. was unable to establish new declarative memories about recent events or facts, he was able to retrieve memories about events that occurred in childhood. Such dissociations between access to older memories and the ability to create new memories has been attested in other studies (Russell & Nathan, 1946 cited in Squire & Alvarez, 1995). There are also dissociations between access to older memories and more recently acquired memories in patients, where damage was limited to the hippocampal regions (Rempel-Clower et al. unpublished data cited in Squire and Alvarez, 1995; Rempel-Clower, Zola, Squire, & Amaral, 1996). In these cases, loss of access to memory is more severe for newer memories and less severe for older memories. This is a pattern that is also confirmed by animal studies in which greater control of the lesion size and time intervals was possible (e.g., Cho, Beracochea, & Jaffard, 1993; Kim & Fanselow, 1992; Squire, 1992; Zola-Morgan & Squire, 1990). These dissociations have been taken as evidence that the stability of memories is temporally dependent and that older declarative memories eventually become dependent on cortical structures and thus would be unaffected by any damage to the hippocampal regions and immediately surrounding cortex.

In recent years, the Standard Theory has been reexamined. Experimental evidence challenges the assertion that older consolidated memories are not as susceptible to disruption. Recent studies (e.g., Miller & Matzel, 2000; Millin, Moody, & Riccio, 2000; Pryzbyslawski & Sara, 1997) and a careful look at older studies (Mactutus, Riccio, & Ferek, 1979; Misanin, Miller, & Lewis, 1968) have shown that memories that are "reactivated," or recalled, may be as vulnerable as newly formed memories. Additionally, Nadel and Moscovitch (1997) provided evidence that the hippocampus is still involved in the retrieval of older episodic and spatial memories. They propose a new theory, *the multiple trace theory*, which challenges the long held belief that long-term memories are eventually established in the neocortex with no connection to the hippocampus.

Multiple Trace Theory

Nadel and Moscovitch (1997) claimed that long-term episodic and spatial memories depend on the hippocampal formation for an indefinite period of time. Multiple Trace Theory and the Standard Theory agree that the initial consolidation of a memory occurs when input from the cortex is sent to the hippocampus and a memory trace is established. MTT and Standard Consolidation theory diverge when explaining how the memory is stabilized over time. Nadel and Moscovich (1997, 1998) asserted that the connections between the hippocampus and the cortical regions are maintained and sometimes strengthened over time through the establishment of multiple traces that are indexed to diverse areas in the cortex.

Figure 5.1, modified from Nadel and Moscovitch (1998), illustrates the differences in how the Standard Theory and MTT explain the relationship between the hippocampus and cortex in memory consolidation. As is shown in Fig. 5.1a and c, information related to the memory comes from the neocortex into the hippocampus. In the hippocampus, a trace is made and that trace is indexed to a cortical region. That cortical region, in turn, interacts with other cortical regions. In this stage, the Standard Model (seen in Fig. 5.1a) and the MTT (seen in Fig. 5.1c) agree. As time passes, according to the Standard Model, the links to the hippocampus disappear and final storage of the memory is in the cortex as is shown in Fig. 5.1b. On the other hand, Nadel and Moscovitch (1998) claimed, that as memories are retrieved and rehearsed, multiple traces are made in the hippocampus as is shown in Fig. 5.1d. These traces are indexed to locations in the neocortex. Each time a new set of hippocampal traces is made they are also indexed to the cortex. Thus, each time a memory is rehearsed, previously linked cortical regions would be linked to another set of traces. Additionally, as more associations are made, new cortical regions could be added to the total set of traces for the given memory. Thus, there is a continuous connection between the neocortex and the hippocampus (Nadel & Moscovitch, 1997).

Nadel and Moscovitch (1998) did, however, make a distinction in terms of the final location of memory storage for episodic and semantic memories. They asserted that episodic memories always will involve the hippocampus, whether they are very old memories or newer memories (Nadel & Moscovitch, 1998). Semantic memories, on the other hand, can eventually be stabilized solely in the neocortex. They believe this difference is due to the fact that episodic memories are dependent on contextual or spatial information and semantic memories are not. The hippocampus has been shown to be necessary for contextual and spatial information (e.g., Nadel, 1990; Nadel & Willner, 1980). For episodic memories and spatial memories (subtypes of declarative memory), which require contextual cues, the contextual information in the hippocampus will be activated every time the memory is reactivated. Although semantic memories may not eventually depend on the hippocampus, the process of stabilization, as described by the MTT, will be relevant to learning. This is discussed in more depth later in the chapter.

Nadel and Moscovitch (1997, 1998) supported their theory by reanalyzing amnesia studies. They observed that degradation of memories for personal

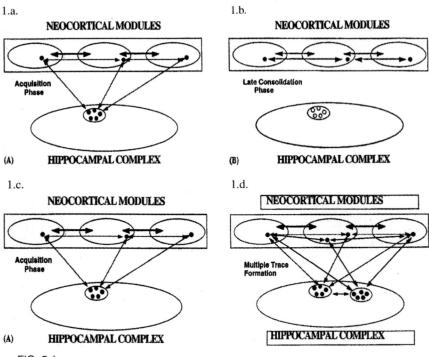

FIG. 5.1.
Standard Theory
1.a. Early Consolidation
1.b. Late Consolidation
     Multiple Trace Theory
1.c. Early Consolidation
1.d. Late Consolidation
Reprinted with adaption from *Neuropharmacology, Vol. 37*, Nadel, L., &
Moscovitch, M., Hippocampal contributions to cortical plasticity, 431–439.
Copyright ©1998, with permission from Elsevier.

events (episodic memory) can extend back as far as 40 years (in a range of
15-40 years). They believe that such an observation questions the notion that
older memories are better preserved than newer memories. Furthermore, there
was a difference in the degree of degradation of autobiographical memories
(episodic) and memories for public events and faces and personal facts (semantic memory). This observation supports their assertion that episodic memories, which are dependent on contextual and spatial cues stored in the
hippocampus, would be more severely damaged by hippocampal damage.

With their colleagues (Nadel, Samsonovich, Ryan, & Moscovitch, 2000), they gave further theoretical and experimental support. In a study of patients with unilateral temporal lobectomy (Viskontas, McAndrews, & Moscovitch, 2000, cited in Nadel et al., 2000), Viskontas et al. found that patients had retrograde amnesia for autobiographical events that went back to early childhood. They asserted that it would be unlikely that the temporary consolidation process as proposed by the Standard Theory should last so long. In another study (Moscovitch, Yaschyshyn, Ziegler, & Nadel, 1999), the authors found that written descriptions of personal episodes were significantly less detailed than those of normal controls. There was a 50% difference between the controls and the amnesic patients in terms of the level of detail. This shows that, whereas the amnesics may have access to the main idea of the events, they have lost many of the contextual details of the episodic memory. In an fMRI study (Ryan et al., 2000), the authors found that the hippocampus was activated when the subjects recalled remote memories—even those 20 to 40 years old.

In summary, the findings in these studies indicate that the loss of episodic memories due to damage to the hippocampus is not limited to just newer memories as claimed by the Standard Theory. Because degradation of episodic memories can extend as far back as 40 years, this suggests, as the proponents of the MTT claim, that the hippocampus must be involved in the storage and retrieval of episodic memories. Table 5.2 summarizes the differences between the MTT and the standard theory.

TABLE 5.2
Summary of Major Claims of the Standard Theory
of Consolidation and MTT

Stage of Consolidation	Standard Theory		MTT	
	Area	Process	Area	Process
Initial Formation of Memory	Hippocampus	Molecular changes (LTP, protein synthesis)	Hippocampus	Molecular changes (LTP, protein synthesis)
Strengthening of memory over time	Hippocampus & Cortical regions	Weakening traces Strengthening traces	Hippocampus & Cortical regions	Multiple traces in hippocampus indexed to areas in the cortex
Stabilization of memory: Episodic/ Spatial	Cortical regions	No traces in hippocampus Strong cortical activity	Hippocampus & Cortex	Cortical regions activate spatial and contextual traces in hippocampus
Stabilization of memory: Semantic	Cortical regions	No traces in hippocampus Strong cortical activity	Cortical Regions	Links to contextual traces in the hippocampus can be lost

One might notice that the MTT does claim that semantic memory can eventually be stabilized in the cortex, which is similar to what the Standard Theory claims about all types of memory. However, there are two reasons to prefer the MTT to the Standard Theory as the basis for a theory of lexical learning. First, in choosing a biological theory, we want a theory that accounts for all types of learning. Both the Standard Theory and MTT explain semantic learning, but the MTT can also account for episodic memories, as well as, other types of hippocampal dependent memory. Secondly, as is explained in more depth later in the chapter, how memory is retrieved is an important concept in explaining how language is stored. When the lexical items are first memorized, the traces and the contextual information can be relevant to lexical learning. MTT can incorporate retrieval in explaining language whereas the Standard Theory cannot. It is preferable not to posit two theories for learning—one for establishing information in memory and one for retrieval of information, which Standard Theory would require us to do. Thus, the MTT has more explanatory power.

Further support for the MTT comes from the finding that older reactivated memories can be disrupted by the methods that also disrupt newly formed memories. This discussion introduces the importance of the role of retrieval in understanding the stability of long-term memories, and this is particularly important in explaining access to lexical items. The fact that experimental cues can make older memories susceptible to disruption goes against the premise of traditional consolidation theory (Miller & Matzel, 2000). Miller and Matzel (2000) asserted that it is not only temporal duration, but also the state of a memory (i.e., whether it has been activated or not) that can affect the stability of the memory. This is a feature of memory that Standard Theory cannot account for but MTT can. MTT emphasizes that memories can be strengthened by repeated retrieval, so accessing memory is as important to its stability as time is.

Several studies provide evidence that certain experimental interventions can interfere not only with initial memory consolidation but also with older consolidated memories during retrieval (Miller & Matzel, 2000; Millin et al., 2000; Pryzbyslawski & Sara, 1997). In all of these experiments, an animal is trained in a task; the day after it has been trained, a substance or condition that can disrupt memory is administered. These experimental treatments (e.g., electroconvulsive shock, chemical modulators, or extreme cold) can interfere with cellular consolidation. These substances are introduced under two contrasting conditions: A day after training, the animal is given the experimental treatment and then is tested in its ability to perform the task it was trained to do, or a day after training, the animal is presented a contextual cue from the training, which reactivates the episodic memory of learning the task.

Then the animal is subjected to the experimental treatment and tested on its ability to perform the task.

In all cases, the animals who were not presented with a contextual cue before the treatment exhibited no disruption in performance of the task. This is what would be predicted because the cellular changes necessary for the onset of consolidation have already been completed. However, the animals whose memories are reactivated by the contextual cue exhibit an impaired performance in the task. This means that their memory of how to perform the task has been disrupted.

This "experimentally induced amnesia" cannot be explained by the Standard Theory (Miller & Matzel 2000). Interestingly, according to Miller and Matzel, many of these observations were made 30 years ago. Misanin et al. (1968) found that electrical shocks caused retrograde amnesia for the conditioned fear response when administered a day after training with a training cue. Mactutus et al. (1979) observed that both mild and severe hypothermia caused decreased fear conditioning in rats who were presented with a contextual cue from the training before the hypothermia treatment a day after training. Pryzbyslawski and Sara (1997) tested the effects of NMDA receptor antagonists and the performance of animals in test trials of a well-learned spatial task. In their studies, animals were trained on an eight-arm maze in search of food. Once the animals reached the acquisition criterion (3 consecutive days with one error), they were tested on a number of test trials, which included spatial cues from the training sessions. Animals injected with MK-801 (NMDA receptor antagonist) after being shown a contextual cue from the training, showed impaired performance on test trials.

Evidence suggests that like the Multiple Trace Theory, a model of retrieval should be considered. Nader et al. (2000a) also conducted a study of disruptions of fear learning by injecting anisomycin into the lateral amygdala of animals when memories were being reactivated. Injections of anisomycin disrupted the reactivation of older memories in the same way it blocked consolidation of new memories. This demonstrates that memories are susceptible to change when reactivated, suggesting that there may be reconsolidation of traces. According to Nader et al. (2000a), this may support the idea of multiple traces. However, they further asserted that one must maintain a distinction between consolidation (of new traces) and reconsolidation (of reactivated traces). Nader et al. also suggested that there could be a distinct neurobiological marker on cells during the consolidation process, which could distinguish new traces from reconsolidated traces. If such a marker were found, it could offer further support for the MTT.

Millin et al. (2000) also recognized that the traditional consolidation theory is not adequate to explain experimentally induced amnesia and recovery. Experimental evidence suggests that the fragility of memories is "activity dependent" and not just age dependent (Millin et al., 2000). However, they found a theory of simple "reconsolidation" to be equally inadequate. They propose the retrieval-based theory. This theory asserts that "the strength of retrograde amnesia is inversely related to the interval between acquisition/reactivation of target episode and the amnesic manipulation" (p. 69). As is observed with new memories, the susceptibility of a reactivated memory to damage decreases as the length of time between reactivation and the amnesic insult increases. For example, consider two experimental conditions of memory reactivation. In one, the memory is reactivated and a disruptive treatment is applied 5 minutes after reactivation; in the other, the memory is reactivated and the disruptive treatment is applied 60 minutes after reactivation. The damage from the disruptive treatment is worse in the "5 minute condition" than in the "60 minute condition." Furthermore, when comparing consolidation of a new memory to reconsolidation of a reactivated memory, it was found that the time frame in which reactivated memories were susceptible to disruption was shorter than that for new memories. Simply put, Millin et al.'s retrieval-based theory asserts that stability of memories (learned information) is *both* activity and time dependent.

The fragility of memory has also been attested in human studies. Research by Loftus and colleagues showed that episodic memories for events can be altered by postevent information (i.e., new information presented to a subject after an event can affect the way the subject remembers and recalls the event). This can cause the person to add information to their memory report or report information incorrectly (Loftus, Miller, & Burns, 1978). Post-event information can even cause a person to develop a memory for a remote past event that did not happen (false memory) (Loftus & Pickrell, 1995). A recent study (Wright, Loftus, & Hall, 2001) demonstrated that post event information can also inhibit the report of certain details from the original memory.

Thus, in studying lexical learning or finding a model of hippocampal dependent memory formation, one must consider three important factors:

1. The overall age of the memory.
2. The number of times a memory has been reactivated (reactivation strengthens memories).
3. The state of the memory (activated or not activated) in the event of any type of disruption.

The MTT and the complementary retrieval based theories (Miller & Matzel, 2000; Millin et al., 2000; Nader et. al., 2000b) can account for the facts about the memory degradation and can also explain how memories can both be strengthened and disrupted by retrieval.

Summary of Consolidation Theories

In this section, I have reviewed the three major approaches to the study of memory consolidation. Studies in the framework of the molecular consolidation theory provide an in-depth description of the cellular processes involved in consolidation within the hippocampus. How these cellular changes are modified is the focus of study within the modulation-of-consolidation theories. Modulatory influences, particularly from the amygdala, have been found to be important not only in the creation of certain types of memory such as conditioned fear response, but also in strengthening or weakening memories formed through other memory systems. The study of the systems themselves is the focus of the neuropsychological theories. In particular, I compared the Standard Consolidation Theory and the Multiple Trace Theory and argued that the MTT is a better model for memory consolidation. The MTT also emphasizes the importance of retrieval in memory formation. Although this discussion emphasizes a neuropsychological model for language learning, it is important to remember that neuropsychological models such as MTT are fundamentally modeling integrated neural circuits, which include cellular processes. Furthermore, these systems themselves are subject to modulation by nonmemory systems. In the next section, I discuss how MTT and the related retrieval-based theories can explain lexical processing in the first language and language learning in second language acquisition.

NEUROBIOLOGICAL THEORY OF LEXICAL LEARNING

I now show the implications of MTT for lexical learning by demonstrating that MTT is compatible with neurally based language theories, particularly Ullman, et al.'s (1997) declarative/procedural model and Pulvermüller's (1999) Hebbian Model of Language (HML). This section addresses the importance of cortical and hippocampal networks to building the lexicon in both first and second language. The declarative/procedural model and the HML are both based primarily on evidence from first language lexicon use, but these theories are shown to be applicable to second language lexical learning. In the next section, I address how MTT and HML might explain some of the characteristics of adult second language acquisition. From this discussion, I conclude that although particular cortical areas do show a dominance for certain kinds of lexical items, lexical processing is supported by a dynamic, integrated neural network—one not specialized for language, but rather one that also functions for memory formation.

The Lexicon: Declarative/Procedural Model

Ullman et al.'s (1997) declarative/procedural model demonstrates that lexical items of different types may be represented in different cortical regions and that the declarative memory system participates in lexical processing. Ullman et al. (1997) present a dual model for language in which they posit that the lexicon is processed by the declarative memory system and grammar is processed by the procedural memory system. According to their model, the neural substrates for the procedural memory system are the frontal cortex and the basal ganglia whereas the declarative memory system is identified as the temporal lobe, including the medial temporal lobe structures such as the hippocampus. Their model is based on the use of irregular and regular verbs. According to their theory, irregular verbs, which must be memorized, are processed by the declarative memory system. Regular verbs, which are rule based, are processed by the procedural memory system.

Ullman et al. (1997) tested the abilities of five patient groups to use a verb (regular, irregular or nonword) in a sentence context. These groups were Alzheimer's patients, anterior aphasics, posterior aphasics, Parkinson's patients, and Huntington's patients. Anterior aphasics were those subjects who had damage predominantly to the frontal regions (including Broca's area) and regions within the basal ganglia. Posterior aphasics had damage predominantly to occipito-parietal areas including the supramarginal gyrus, angular gyrus, superior parietal lobule, occipital areas involved in vision (Brodmann's Areas 18, 19) and Wernicke's area. Classically, anterior aphasics are considered to be agrammatic, whereas posterior aphasics generally have lexical or semantic impairments. Thus, the anterior aphasics were predicted to have impairments with regular verbs, but not irregular verbs, whereas posterior aphasics would have trouble with irregular verbs, but not regular verbs. Alzheimer's patients have impairments in forming new memories and accessing older declarative memories; they were predicted to have more difficulties with irregular verbs, than with regular verbs. Parkinson's and Huntington's patients, on the other hand, have degeneration in the basal ganglia, which is the primary neural substrate for procedural memory. Thus, they were predicted to have greater difficulty with regular verbs than irregular verbs.

As predicted, the Alzheimer's patients and posterior aphasics exhibited problems with irregular verbs, whereas the anterior aphasics, Parkinson's and Huntington's patients had trouble inflecting regular verbs. These findings support the assertion that impairments in the declarative memory system can cause impairments in the access to lexical items, in this case, the memorized forms of irregular verbs. Ullman (2001a) offered further evidence from neuroimaging studies (PET, fMRI, and ERP), which confirms that lexical and semantic processing is associated with temporal lobe activation and that syntactic processing is associated with basal ganglia and frontal lobe activation (specifically, Broca's area and the supplementary motor area).

Sonnenstuhl, Eisenbeiss, and Clahsen (1999) and Waksler (1999) provide cross-linguistic support for the declarative/procedural model. Sonnenstuhl et al. (1999) found results similar to Ullman (2001a) in native German speakers. Waksler (1999) confirmed the same contrast between regular and irregular verbs in a number of languages from different language families (e.g., Armenian, Cebuano, Chinese, German, Hebrew, Hungarian, Indonesian, Korean, Russian, Swedish, Tagalog, and Urdu).

The declarative/procedural model provides evidence that the processing of verb forms (memorized as lexical items) depends on the declarative memory system and thus can be related to the MTT. However, because the evidence for the declarative/procedural model largely comes from the studies of adults and children who have already acquired language, Ullman et al.'s studies themselves provide no information on the processes involved as lexical items are being learned. Synthesizing the MTT with the declarative/procedural model can offer insight to the underlying neural processes when lexical items are first being learned or how the memories for the lexical items might be processed. To date, few, if any imaging studies have been conducted on subjects learning second language vocabulary, *as they are learning the vocabulary* for the first time. Studies may require a subject to learn lists or groups of words for a task, but these are usually words that the person is already familiar with. Thus, although we know from imaging studies that lexical processing involves the hippocampal regions (medial temporal regions), researchers have not yet confirmed or studied the involvement of the hippocampal regions in initial learning of lexical items. However, from our understanding of memory development in MTT, it can be inferred that the processes involved in memory consolidation are involved in word learning, particularly in the very early stages. The MTT offers a guide of what kind of studies of early vocabulary learning can be done. In the next section, I review another model of language learning, the Hebbian Model of Language. The examination of this model further confirms the usefulness of using a memory theory to constrain the study of neuro-biological theories of lexical learning.

The Lexicon: Hebbian Model of Language (HML) and MTT

Pulvermüller's Hebbian Model of Language (1999) provided a neuronal expla-nation of lexical development supporting the idea that neural substrates for lexi-cal items are not dedicated local circuits, but rather widely dispersed cortical networks—networks also posited by MTT. Pulvermüller's theory focuses pri-marily on cortical networks and measures how they work for adults who have al-ready acquired lexical items; integrating the MTT with the HML shows how these cortical networks might first be established through a connection with the hippocampus, including how the semantic memories in the cortical regions might first be established.

Pulvermüller (1999) based his HML on the cell assembly model of Hebb (1949). Hebb's (1949) notion of cell assemblies states that neurons that fire to-gether can become associated and act as a single functional unit called a *cell as-sembly* (see also chap. 4). These cell assemblies can consist of neurons that are close or distant, thus making it possible for cognitive functions to be repre-sented by a dispersed set of neurons. Pulvermüller briefly described how these cell assemblies could be established for lexical items. When a word is being learned, a learner receives a variety of information about the word: the form, the meaning (semantics), its morphosyntactic features, how it is used in con-text, and its pronunciation. All this information, which may have its origins in different cortical locations, can be represented by a widely dispersed cortical network. Furthermore, even when one considers one subset of information, for example, semantics, information still comes from a variety of sources. In the case of semantics, stimuli from all of the modalities related to the word is in-cluded in the cell assembly. These features may include color, shape, move-ment, form, animacy or inanimacy.

From his own studies and a review of major lexical studies, Pulvermüller described where the processing of lexical items may be occur. In EEG and MEG studies, Pulvermüller found that there is a distinction between where function words (e.g., grammatical morphemes, articles, etc.) and content words are processed. The processing of function words is strongly lateralized to the left hemisphere whereas content words are less strongly lateralized (Neville, Mills, & Lawson, 1992; Pulvermüller, Lutzenberger, & Birbaumer, 1995; Pulvermüller & Mohr, 1996). Pulvermüller believed this fits the cell assembly interpretation. Because function words have fewer semantic associations, there would be fewer cortical associations among the sensory regions of the cortex.

Using ERP, Pulvermüller demonstrates further, that content words are processed in cortical areas that are related to the features of the lexical items. Pulvermüller, Lutzenberger, and Preissl (1999) studied the distinction between action and visual associated content words. In these cases, a motor action or a visual image respectively may be associated with the word. Action words (words which have a strong movement component associated with them) were processed in the perisylvian areas and motor cortices. Words that are visually perceived were processed in the perisylvian areas (middle temporal gyrus) and the occipital regions near the primary visual area (Damasio, Grabowski, Tranel, & Hichwa, 1996; Pulvermüller, 1999).

Other lexical studies support this idea. In their review paper, Martin and Chao (2001) found that lexical items were processed in the areas associated with the semantic features of the words. Thus, words representing object motion were processed in the lateral middle temporal gyrus, an area that processes the actual perception of motion (Bonda, Petrides, Ostry, & Evans, 1996; Puce, Allison, Bentin, Gore, & McCarthy, 1998). Furthermore, words, such as those for tools, with use-associated meanings were processed in the ventral premotor cortex. Based on findings from Hoshi and Tanji (2000), Martin and Chao (2001) suggested that this reflects the fact that this region is also responsible for action planning.

Nouns seem to be associated with the ventral-occipito-temporal cortex (Chao, Haxby, & Martin, 1999; Martin, Wiggs, Ungerleider, & Haxby, 1996; Perani et al., 1995, 1999). This area is part of the ventral visual pathway (see chap. 6 for another discussion of the relevance of this area) and is an area that Martin and Chao (2001) see as a feature space. They call this region a feature space because words processed here are those concrete nouns with no motor or movement associations but rather have associations based on other features. These features may have to do with animacy or inanimacy (Caramazza & Shelton, 1998), color (Chao & Martin, 1999) or being a naturally occurring or man-made object (Kreiman, Koch, & Fried, 2000; Moore & Price, 1999 cited in Martin & Chao, 2001). Martin and Chao (2001) reject the idea that the ventral-occipito-temporal cortex consists of subareas specifically dedicated to specific word categories (i.e., an area specifically for color words, another for furniture or houses, etc.). Rather it is more important to consider the representation of features because many words may fall into a number of word categories. Thus, Martin and Chao (2001) have demonstrated that brain areas involved in the processing of words are areas that also process nonlinguistic information that is related to the features of the words. These findings are consistent with Pulvermüller's (1999) finding that concrete nouns (which are visually perceived) are processed in the middle temporal region and the occipital cortex.

Pulvermüller and his colleagues discovered that the feature-specific location of lexical processing can be quite specific. Pulvermüller, Haerle and Hummel (2000, 2001) compared the processing of the three types of words in German: verbs related to leg movement (*to jump*), verbs related to arm movement (*to lift*) and verbs related to the face or mouth (*to kiss*). Using EEG recordings, they found that leg related words showed activation in areas along the medial motor strip where leg movement is processed. Likewise, arm and mouth/face related words showed activation in lateral areas that process arm and face movement.

Thus far, I have discussed the evidence for where the processing of lexical items takes place and how this evidence supports the HML. The dispersed cortical locations for processing are consistent with a dispersed cortical cell assembly. An increase in activity when words are compared to pseudowords provides evidence that this dispersed cortical activity is indeed related to word processing (Pulvermüller & Mohr, 1996).

The cortical cell assembly theory relates closely to the MTT. The MTT emphasizes that there is an ongoing connection between the hippocampus and the cortical areas during learning. Although this connection remains only for episodic learning after the memory is well-established, it is present for semantic memories in the initial stages and intermediate stages of semantic learning. I address two consequences of this feature in regard to lexical learning: the sites for lexical storage and processing, and the role contextual cues can have in strengthening lexical learning.

According to the MTT, when a word is first learned both the contextual and semantic features that are associated with the word are included in the memory (Nadel & Moscovitch, 1997). Take, for example, an instance when a word is being learned. Information about the lexical items would come from multiple sensory areas. If presented visually, information would come into the hippocampus from the temporal and occipital areas (Kaas & Hackett, 1999; Romanski , Tian, Fritz, Goldman-Rakic, & Rauschecker, 1999). Additionally, information about the word's pronunciation, its meaning, and its grammatical classification may come in from other cortical areas. In the hippocampus, traces would be laid down. Initially, the contextual cues from the learning environment may be included in the traces for the lexical item. This information then is sent back, minimally, to the cortical areas from which the information came (Chrobak et al., 2000). Cortical-cortical connections (cell assemblies) between the original cortical areas can then be made, as described by Pulvermueller and discussed earlier. The hippocampus continues to interact over time with these areas via the cortical-hippocampal connections. While the lexical item is being learned, each time the memory of the lexical item is activated, new traces will be laid down in the hippocampus and indexed to the cortical regions. This resonates with Hebb's Law, namely that reactivation results in a strongly connected set of neurons (i.e., cell assembly). As the lexical item is used in new situations, new associations are made between the hippocampus and new cortical regions. Eventually, the memory becomes separated from the original contextual cues and become consolidated in the cortical areas. Pulvermueller's HML only addresses the cortico-cortical relationships. Because the MTT also models the relationship between the cortex and the hippocampus, it can offer a more comprehensive model of lexical learning than HML alone.

So, even if lexical items become stabilized in the cortex, the areas in which they are stabilized are the sensory areas associated with the initial information about the word that was sent to the hippocampus. It seems, therefore, that the eventual locations of the lexical items are the areas associated with either: the modality of input or the features of the lexical items. In summary, lexical processing is supported by a dispersed network of connections between hippocampal structures and areas of cortex that may show dominance for processing lexical items with certain features or functions.

Neurobiological Lexical Theories and MTT: Conclusion

In this first section, I discussed Ullman's declarative/procedural model of language and Pulvermüller's HML and showed how these neurobiological theories are compatible with the memory model, MTT. Their compatibility supports the MTT's usefulness as a lexical learning model. Ullman's model substantiates the validity of applying a declarative memory model such as MTT to language learning. The HML provides a model detailing cortical representation of the lexicon, which fits the relationship between the cortical regions and the hippocampus as described by the MTT. As stated earlier, both the declarative/procedural model and HML only address the location of lexical items after they are acquired. Ullman's (2001b) recent work has shown that this model appropriately predicts the characteristics of second language grammar and lexicon, but still does not provide a full systematic description of the role of the hippocampus early in acquisition. The MTT can provide a comprehensive neurobiological system accounting for lexical items as they are being learned and after they are consolidated.

In the next section, I apply the MTT to second language acquisition scenarios in order to show how, theoretically, MTT could explain some of the characteristics of adult second language acquisition. A hypothetical application of the theories can also serve to assess the explanatory power of this model for language acquisition and help us develop testable research questions. Two aspects of second language acquisition make it a good candidate to serve as a test case for a neurobiological theory of lexical learning. First, the language of adult second language learners is testable by imaging techniques. Imaging young children, although possible, is much more difficult. Imaging is not the only a viable means for measuring neurological involvement in language, but has the advantage of providing on-line measures of activity. Furthermore, differences in processing observed between the first and second language could make possible the generation of inferences about first language acquisition. Secondly, the significant individual differences in anatomical location of the second language and individual differences in proficiency among second language speakers, not seen to the same degree in normal first language learners, make it a good candidate to test the hypothesis that the MTT can serve as a model of the mechanism for lexical learning (Ellis, 1994; Genesee, 1988).

SECOND LANGUAGE LEXICON

There are a number of advantages to explaining lexical learning through a theory such as MTT. It is more parsimonious to have one mechanism for learning than to have to posit a learning mechanism for spatial learning, episodic learning, learning of general facts about the world and then another just for learning language features. This is particularly true because it can be shown that aspects of language learning have features that make them likely to be just like other types of learning (e.g., information comes from sensory areas, usually auditory and visual). These findings suggest that all of the elements necessary for learning a lexical item are already available in non-language specific neural systems. There are no special mechanisms or special places for lexical items per se. As these findings seem to indicate, words do not seem to group together by the fact that they are words; they are more likely to be located in places that are associated with sensory features, or object features, or by factors involved in acquisition. Thus, there seems to be no natural neurobiological grouping of lexical items in general.

Similar ideas have been advocated by Paradis (1997) who argued that the neural bases of two languages in bilinguals are not necessarily anatomically distinct even if in some cases they are functionally distinct. There has been considerable debate and uncertainty about the state of the bilingual lexicon (Kroll & de Groot, 1997; Smith, 1997). Cognitive theories have proposed that the two lexicons are completely distinct, whereas others see them as distinct only in terms of lexical forms but not semantic concepts (Kroll & de Groot, 1997). The major models of the bilingual lexicon, as reviewed by Lotto and de Groot (1998), include the word-association model and concept mediation model of Potter, So, Von Eckardt, and Feldman (1984) and the picture association model of Chen (1990). The word association model states that concepts that underlie lexical semantics must be accessed through the lexicon of the first language. In concept mediation, the L1 and L2 lexicons are distinct but each has direct access to concepts. In the picture association model, the L1 lexicon has direct access to concepts whereas the L2 has access to concepts only through images, that is, if an L2 learner is shown a word in the L2, he or she will not directly access a concept related to that word. However, if he or she is shown a picture that he or she must label in the L2, the learner can access the concept because he or she has a concept related to the picture.

The neurobiological memory theory, MTT, and the Hebbian Model of Language offer a new perspective on the lexicon. In the recent literature, the lexicon in each language is referred to as a *separate store*. The lexicons can be seen as distinct from each other and, as is seen in the previously mentioned models, the L2 lexicon itself can be disconnected from the conceptual level. The current ways of looking at the lexicon imply that lexical items in the L1 will be strongly associated with each other. Furthermore, lexical items in the L2, by virture of fact that they are all words in the L2, will be strongly associated with each other. However, both the MTT and Hebbian model of language show that when a particular lexical item is being processed, the information about linguistic form (phonological information), semantics, word features, and associated concepts is activated together. Therefore, if an item in L1 and L2 share similar word features (color, animacy, motor associations), it is possible that they will have similar activations. Furthermore, based on the neurobiological theories, it seems that concepts may be a part of the cell assembly network that is activated when a word is being processed. Certainly, I do not presume that the word association, concept mediation, and picture association models are proposing that the L1 and L2 lexicons have specific anatomical locations. Nevertheless, I think it may be misleading even to think of all of the L1 lexicon as being separable from all of the L2 lexicon.

Individual Differences: Location

In neurological terms, it has been difficult to locate the lexicon. Cortical-stimulation studies (Ojemann & Whitaker, 1978) indicate that the bilingual lexicon is widely distributed. The cortical stimulation procedures were done on two patients prior to temporal lobectomy surgery. Twenty-three stimulation sites on the cortex were selected at the beginning of the operation. The patient was then shown a series of black and white line drawings of common objects and the phrase, "This is a " written above the picture. As the picture of the object first appeared, stimulation of one of the sites began. At the same time, the patient would respond to the prompt. Ojemann and Whitaker demonstrated that a single stimulation of a site may affect both languages. Other cortical sites, on the other hand, affect only one of the languages. Figure 5.2, taken from Fabrro's (1999) adaptation of Ojemann and Whitaker (1978) shows the location of lexical processing for two languages. Such inhomogeneity in the location of lexicons across individuals would not be unexpected on an MTT account. Because the features of the lexicons are different and learners use different strategies, the indexing of information would be distributed differently for the two languages and across subjects.

It may be that the differential way that the lexicons of the two languages are laid down is a result of the different semantic features associated with the lexical items in the two languages. Such an explanation for first language was asserted by Fuster (1999), in his reply to Pulvermüller's HML (1999); he emphasized that variation in neural substrates for an individual's lexicon is related to the fact that learning the semantic properties of words depends on individual experience. This could occur in second language learning, for instance, in cases where words in one language have broader connotations than their counterpart in another language. Some examples comparing English with a number of languages illustrate the point. The word, *Gemütlichkeit* in German is translated as *hospitality* in English, but it also includes the sense of comfort, well-being, and feeling at home. A number of lexical items in Thai also exemplify this pattern. *Geng*, which is translated as *clever*, can also mean smart, intelligent, knowledgeable, and proficient. *Riebroy*, usually translated as *proper* includes the meanings of being proper, good and appropriate (for people), and clean and well kept (for things).

Another feature of lexical learning, which may account for the different anatomical locations of two languages, is learner strategies. A second language learner may make associations with the mother tongue when learning the

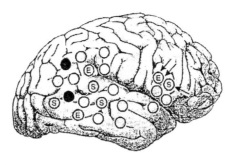

English and Spanish

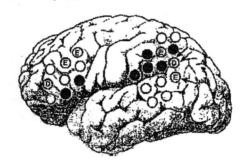

English and Dutch

FIG. 5.2.
English and Spanish
English and Dutch
Reprinted from Fabbro (1999) with permission of authors and publisher of the original figure as it appeared in Ojemann, G. A., & Whitaker, H. A. (1978), The bilingual brain. *Archives of Neurology, 35,* 409–412. Copyright © 1978, American Medical Association. All rights reserved.

word. These associations could involve matching the target word with a semantically similar word in the native language. This could be the case if a learner uses translation as a strategy (for instance, Arabic *sayaara* learned through dependence on the translation, *car*) or if the word is a cognate (French *bleu* [blue]) or a near cognate (German *Sonnenschein* [sunshine]); Arabic *suker* [sugar]).

On the other hand, the strategy could involve associating the target with a semantically different word that is similar to the native language in some other aspect. Such a strategy might be employed by a language learner to make a foreign lexical item more salient and therefore, memorable. The similarity could be phonological—Arabic *barq* (lightning), which sounds similar to English *bark*; Thai *gai* (chicken), which sounds similar to *guy*, or it could be that the word is a false cognate—German *Gift* (poison); Thai *moo* (pig/pork).

The anatomical substrates for the second language lexicon may also be influenced by the differential experience of the learners (Paradis, 1997). Adult second language learners often use learning strategies that may not be used for first language, particularly if the second language is learned in a classroom and contextual cues are used to help with learning (Littlewood, 1994). For example, the cortical location for processing and storing lexical items may differ if the person learned in a classroom and used contextual clues from that room to help with learning the words. In this case, spatial and contextual traces will be strongly linked to the cortical regions in a way that would make these cortical regions active as part of the representation. Furthermore, a classroom learner may also make kinesthetic or visual associations if pictures or movement are used when the words are used. In classroom settings, activities involving movement and word learning are often used to enhance student learning and participation (Krashen, 1995). To illustrate, a teacher may have students follow commands using the words they are learning. He or she might give the students commands such as, "Pick up the *blue* pen. Point to the *yellow* notebook. Put the *blue* pen on a *green* chair. Touch something *black*." Kinetic movement is often even more relevant for an adult learner who is not in a classroom. A learner may make strong movement associations with the words if he or she is in an active work environment ("Give me the pliers." "Turn the stove on." "Get another red tray.") or if gestures are used to facilitate meaning. In the case where color words are associated with movement, we may see activation not only in areas for color perception (V4 of occipital lobe, Zeki, 1993) but also in areas for movement (middle temporal gyrus). Another influential factor is the emotional environment that is associated with the learning of that lexical item. This could include anxiety, stress, culture shock, embarrassment, or any positive emotions (Ellis, 1994; Larsen-Freeman & Long, 1991; Littlewood, 1994; Skehan, 1989).

Individual Differences in Proficiency: The Role of Spatial and Contextual Cues, and Rehearsal

These learner strategies may also be relevant to the individual differences in proficiency among adult second language learners. Strategies such as making associations with the first language, using kinesthetic, visual, or contextual cues, and rehearsal can affect whether a word is well-learned or not. Individual variation in language proficiency among second language learners is often substantial and is one of the distinguishing factors between first and second language learning. MTT can explain not only the vast differences in the location of the bilingual or second language lexicon, but can explain differences in individuals' abilities to remember words in the second language. Access to traces for contextual cues can have an effect on how extensive the neural network for a particular lexical item is. Let us now look at an example of how using contextual clues could aid learning and retention of a lexical item. Although the hippocampus may not be crucial for access to lexical items after words have been well learned, it is involved when the words are being memorized (Kohler, Moscovitch, Wincour, & McIntosh, 2000). According to the MTT, when a word is first learned (i.e., a semantic memory is established), both the contextual and semantic features that are associated with the words are laid down in traces in the hippocampus (Nadel & Moscovitch, 1997). Therefore, initially, there are traces for the contextual information. Contextual information would be relevant to a student learning words in a classroom situation. Traces for the semantic features of the word, the contextual information from the classroom, other students in the classroom and any spatial information would be encoded.

As previously stated, when the memory traces are laid down, contextual cues can be included. The contextual cues could aid in the memory of the word and might even be linked to visual cues or kinetic movement (spatial cues) associated with it. As the word is rehearsed, the contextual cues are rehearsed with it. So, these cues, which augment the meaning of the word, will be activated each time, perhaps helping the learner use the word.

There are two ways that the presence of these traces during learning could explain whether or not this word would be well learned. It could be that with time, the contextual cues are lost, but their presence at the time of learning helps the word become more salient in the mind of the learner. This greater saliency is due to the greater cortical activation in the cell assembly. These connections have been established through indexing with the hippocampal traces during learning. Even after the connections with the hippocampus are lost, the cortical-cortical connections would remain. It could also be that, for this word, the contextual or spatial cues are never lost, although over time their presence may be reduced. Thus, the person always has cues to aid in the retrieval of the features of the words. Such methods of learning words may be unusual in people learning the lexicon in their first language, but they are frequently used by people learning a second language. This is just one example of a strategy employed for lexical learning in a second language. Similar logic could be applied to other commonly used second language learner strategies: translation, grouping, imagery, auditory representation, direct or physical response (Ellis, 1994), repetition and rehearsal.

These principles can have explanatory power beyond lexical learning. As mentioned at the outset of this chapter, the mechanisms of memory formation should not just be seen as a lexical learning mechanism, but also as a mechanism for all aspects of adult second language learning such as learning grammatical rules. One aspect of adult second language learning that has been notably different from first language learning is the failure of most adult second language learners to become completely proficient. Fossilization and a lack of complete proficiency have been a well-studied phenomenon (see Ellis, 1994; see also Lee, chap. 3 & Schuchert, chap. 6, for further discussion). I now briefly address how the memory theories discussed in this chapter might be relevant.

One impediment to complete proficiency that has been identified extensively in SLA literature is anxiety. As was mentioned earlier, the state of a memory is important to the strength of its consolidation. It has been shown in animal studies that reactivated memories can be disturbed by experimental interventions (Mactutus et al., 1979; Miller & Matzel, 2000; Millin et al., 2000; Misanin et al., 1968; Pryzbyslawski & Sara, 1997). I would like to suggest that analogous disruptions in real life situations (stress, anxiety, competing information) could also disrupt the consolidation of lexical items if these interrupting factors occur when the lexical item or grammatical rule is being rehearsed or retrieved. So, in the same way rehearsal could increase the stability of a memory for a particular lexical item or grammatical rule, disruptions during rehearsal could cause extinction or degradation of the memory for the lexical item. A full exploration of the topic is not pursued here. My goal here is to make an initial suggestion. But to fully understand the applicability of the MTT to understanding disruptions in language learning, a careful study of the anxiety and stress in SLA literature must be done. What should be clear is that the MTT theory has potential for providing a mechanism that can explain many characteristics of adult second language learning.

BEYOND THE LEXICON: APHASIA IN ADULT SECOND LANGUAGE LEARNERS AND OTHER BILINGUALS

So far, this chapter has focused on how the memory theory, MTT, considered with the lexical theories, can provide a neural mechanism for lexical learning and how MTT may also explain other features of the language of adult second language learners, or late bilinguals. What has not yet been addressed is the applicability of this neural mechanism to other types of bilinguals (such as early bilinguals, who learn multiple languages before the onset of puberty). Studies by Ullman and colleagues (1997; 2001a, b), discussed earlier in this paper, have shown that second language learners will more likely have both grammar and lexicon supported by the declarative memory system (temporal lobe), whereas first language learners' grammar will be supported by the procedural memory system (frontal lobe and basal ganglia) and only the lexicon may be supported by the temporal lobe system. Furthermore, early bilinguals, who are proficient, will pattern more like first language learners. Kim, Relkin, Lee, and Hirsch (1997) also found, in their fMRI study, that late second language learners represented their first and second language differently than early bilinguals. This seems to suggest that the MTT might only be applicable to adult second language learners. I show, however, that MTT can apply to a range of bilingual states and can provide a new way to interpret the recovery patterns in bilingual aphasia.

The status of bilinguals has been hard to categorize since there is great variability among bilinguals. As already seen, bilinguals can vary in terms of time frame of acquisition (pre- or post-puberty), eventual level of proficiency of each language, and the context of acquisition. This has lead to descriptions of bilinguals as being of different types, summarized by Pavlenko (1999) as:

1. Coordinate bilinguals: those who learn their two languages in different environments.
2. Compound bilinguals: those who learn their language in the same environment. These bilinguals also use both languages within the same context.
3. Subordinate bilinguals: those bilinguals who learn the second language later in life. These are bilinguals who can be characterized as second or foreign language learners.

Although these characterizations do broadly describe patterns of cerebral representation and loss of language in bilinguals, studies of individual cases have not been able to support one theory over another. This is a shortcoming noted by Paradis (1997; 1998), who noted that the variability among bilinguals may be due to their variable dependence on the declarative or nondeclarative memory systems. However, to completely understand the role declarative memory plays, we need to indentify the mechanisms of the declarative system and determine how these mechanisms might explain variability among bilinguals. What we will find is that there can never be one theory to explain bilingual learning if this theory is based solely on describing language loss in bilinguals.

The MTT can contribute to our understanding of differing patterns of language loss and recovery in the case of aphasia/anomia. First of all, the MTT may help us understand why languages can be recovered. Many aphasics are able to recover and regain the use of their language. Clearly, this is indicative of a dynamic neural system. For if languages were truly *stored* in places, there should not be any chance of recovery. The MTT explanation is compatible with the Activation Threshold Argument (Paradis, 1998). According to this theory, the trace for a lexical item or rule can be activated once a certain level of neural firing is reached. The more a word or rule is used the lower the threshold level is for activation.

This also relates to another explanation given for aphasic syndromes, namely, that it is not a problem of representation, but a problem of access (Paradis, 1998). In this case, representation of the language itself is not lost, but the ability to access this information is impaired or inhibited. This proposal is compatible with the "reconsolidation" of traces. Reconsolidation may be relevant in a number of recovery situations. Evidence from aphasia studies show that the resulting language impairments due to damage and recovery patterns from this damage vary widely among bilinguals (Fabbro, 1999; Paradis, 1998). Paradis (1998) identified six major recovery patterns in bilingual aphasics: parallel recovery (recovery of all languages at the same rate), selective recovery (one or more of the languages is not recovered at all), successive recovery (one language is recovered fully before any others are recovered), differential recovery (one language has a better recovery than another), antagonistic recovery (one language recovers as another gets worse), and blending (a patient mixes the two languages).

Such differences have been attributed to a number of factors including two classic theories: whether the language was the native language (Ribot, 1881), and which language was most familiar (Pietres, 1895). But, recovery patterns do not fit nicely into these two classic patterns. The concept of reconsolidation of traces, however, can account for these patterns. For example, in the case where a relatively less well used language recovers first, it may be that more traces for the one, less frequently used language are accessible initially. As this language is used, its traces could reactivate traces from other languages through distant associations. In the recovery process, the memories are rebuilt.

Additionally, in his review, Fabbro (1999) identified other factors that can affect the pattern of recovery in bilingual aphasics. These include which language was the most recently used, the orthographic system of the language, emotional factors, the language used in the hospital and the context in which the language was learned and used. Paradis (1997) also noted that the individual experience of a bilingual and the role of declarative versus nondeclarative memory can play an important role in how the languages are organized in the individual brain and how the person might recover from damage. Particularly, Paradis stated that the context of language learning is of crucial importance. This can include whether both languages were learned in a similar environment (i.e., at home) or in two different environments (i.e., at home and at school, or at home and at church).

I have already demonstrated that under the MTT, contextual cues from the learning environment are important in the early stages of memory encoding. Paradis also pointed out the importance of the context of use. Even if both languages may first be learned in the same context, the two languages may not always be used in the same context. There may be patterns of difference: people who learn both languages at home may have similar patterns of impairment and recovery or people who learn one language early at home and the other later in grade school may also have similar patterns of recovery. But, we may also see that, even among people with similar contexts, there may be differences in recovery. In addition to the larger context, we may see the individual's context affecting how their language is stored.

The context of learning may be enough to make learners pattern together in a general sense, but if one looks at individual cases, some individual differences will be seen. Thus, it is important to consider both the macro-level context (e.g., home, school, or work setting) and the micro-level context (individual experience) and the interaction between them. What these previous explanations have captured is the variation in the macro context. What we need to consider is the micro context, or the context of the individual. What the MTT offers is an understanding of the underlying mechanism for how the cortex organizes itself.

The MTT could also offer a systematic neural explanation for why there is such a large array of symptoms among bilinguals. The same concept that applies to episodic memories could apply here. In the case of episodic memories, the concern was for traces in the hippocampus. The older the memory, the more traces there would be in the hippocampus for certain contextual cues. This fact would explain why older episodic memories are less impaired than newer ones (Nadel & Moscovitch, 1998). In the same way, language rules, lexical items, or structures that have been thoroughly rehearsed may have traces that have been stabilized in a number of cortical areas (particularly if the word was related to other words or associated with a number of different features). In this case, a lesion limited to one area of the brain would cause aphasia that was less severe than in a person whose lexicon or language representation had been stabilized in only a few cortical locations. It could also be the case that the differences in the recovery and impairment in bilingual aphasia are related to the differential way in which cortical networks for lexical items or rules are established.

This is particularly interesting in cases when the second language is recovered and the first language is not, and there is no basal ganglia or frontal lesion, which has been shown to be involved in first language representation (Fabbro, 1999; Lee, chap. 3). In such a case one would expect that the first language should be better preserved. If the second language can be recovered, it may be because this language was more widely the dispersed in the cortex, a dispersion due to the network created during acquisition. For example, in the case of M.J., a patient with temporal lobe damage (Halpern, 1941 cited in Fabbro, 1999), he recovered his second language better than his first language. M.J.'s first language was German, but he also used Yiddish at home. M.J. learned literary Hebrew as a teenager, and as an adult used it after moving to Palestine. Yet, after suffering damage to the temporal lobe, he recovered his Hebrew better than his German. This is unexpected because his Hebrew, which was learned after puberty in a school setting, would most likely be dependent on the declarative memory system, which is supported by the temporal lobe region. Another patient, N.K.J., suffered damage to the left temporal-parietal region (Fabbro, 1999). She recovered German, which she learned in high school and studied further at university, but she did not recover speaking ability in her first language, Bulgarian, in which she had been fluent. She had used both Bulgarian and German frequently before her insult. Again, this would not be the pattern expected given that German was learned in school as a teenager and should be supported by the declarative memory system.

These cases exemplify a situation where the macrolevel tells us to expect one pattern, which is not seen at the microlevel. As was shown by Ullman et. al. (1997) and Ullman (2001b), there is clearly a statistical pattern that second language grammar (learned later in life) is supported by the declarative memory system. Yet, when we look at individuals, such as M.J. and N.K.J., we do not see the expected pattern. Such findings are not be totally unexpected when considering the mechanism of declarative memory formation as described in this chapter. According to the MTT, the hippocampus is necessary and active particularly in the early stages of memory formation. But as the memory is rehearsed, connections with other areas of the cerebral cortex are made. The extent of these dispersed networks can vary—but can be very widely distributed in some cases. It could be that these individuals (M.J. and N.K.J.) had widely dispersed representations of their second languages, that could be recovered from traces that were in other areas of the cerebral cortex. This distribution may be due to associations made early in the learning process or associations made in the time before the insult when both individuals used the second language frequently. Why the first language would have been damaged is unclear; a fuller understanding of the relationship between the nondeclarative system would be necessary to explain this. The important point here is that macro level explanations only provide a generalized explanation of group behavior.

Understanding the underlying mechanism of bilingual learning requires looking at the micro or individual level. This does not mean, however, that all patterns of cerebral representation of language are just random. All of the representations of two languages that we may see are the result of the same process. In other words, the mechanism is the same, but this mechanism may lead to different outcomes depending on the conditions during the learning. Theories of linguistic representation that focus on features such as proficiency, context or use, are really theories about the *conditions*, not the underlying unifying mechanism. The unifying features of the representation of two languages in the brain are the neural changes and network building that comprises the individual memory of a language learner.

CONCLUSION

The search for a neurological substrate for language, particularly lexical learning, should not be a search just for "places" in the brain, but rather should attempt to find neural systems which underlie language learning. This chapter has presented the MTT, which is consistent with a possible neurobiological system that could explain lexical learning. It is important to remember that the theories discussed in this chapter are not only relevant to lexical learning. The role of declarative memory consolidation may also relevant to learning grammatical, orthographic, or phonological rules for adult second language learners. The consolidation theory discussed here is the continuation of the cellular processes discussed by Crowell in chapter 4.

So far, I have presented evidence from the memory research and lexical research in first languages. My proposals for second language lexical learning are based on hypothetical examples and an integration of SLA and memory literature. Further research should test the proposals made in this chapter. The first of these is to confirm the role of the hippocampus in second language lexical learning. The hippocampus has been found to be active in verbal encoding, but to date, no study has specifically attempted to test the role of the hippocampus in subjects learning lexical items in a second language. Crowell and I have proposed an fMRI study to test hippocampal activation of native and near-native English speakers' acquisition of Basque. Other proposals made in this chapter also lend themselves to testing by imaging techniques. PET or fMRI studies can determine the location and level of neural activation when learners are using different types of learning strategies, and when a learner is processing words in two languages and the lexical item in one language has greater connotations and broader meanings than the other. Finally, imaging studies could be used to compare the neural activation between proficient and fossilized learners when they are processing lexical items.

6   The Neurobiology of Attention

Sara Ann Schuchert

DEFINING ATTENTION

Introduction

This chapter explores attention research and how attention functions in the brain during learning. Stimuli in the environment are constantly competing for attention and processing resources. Attention is rooted in competition between stimulus-driven behavior and goal-directed response (James, 1950). This constant competition occurs over time and throughout the brain. Stimuli can be external (environmental) or internal (from a learner's own memory or body) (James, 1950). Procedural memory, declarative memory, working memory, and motor planning each play a role in the formation of goals and responses. Memory, goal-directed behavior, stimulus-driven response, and the competition for processing resources all contribute to the creation of "attention." The following pages discuss the neurobiological mechanisms that underlie these aspects of attention. In this chapter visual selective attention, and its role as a model for attention in other modalities (Constantinidis, Williams, & Goldman-Rakic, 2002; James, 1950; Kanwisher & Wojciulik, 2000; Parasuraman, 1998), is drawn on to suggest how the attention process might function in adult second language learning.

Defining Attention

Generally, in discussions about adult second language learning, the word "attention" represents a unitary concept. Historically, attention research has been divided into two (2) categories; attention to salient environmental stimuli, and attention directed by the organism's internal goals (James, 1950). However, like memory, in the current scientific literature, attention is divided into many overlapping categories and subcategories (Parasuraman, 1998). These various sub-categories are useful in that they divide a large, unwieldy topic into parcels small enough to be empirically studied. However, in the literature, definitions of attention and its subcategories are often vague or conflicting. One of the most general definitions argues that attention is voluntary control over automatic brain processes (Posner & Petersen, 1990). This definition gives no neurobiological information and offers only a vague explanation of the attention concept. In more detail, Parasuraman (1998) suggests that attention is comprised of three subcategories: control, vigilance, and selection, all of which permit and maintain goal-directed behavior in the presence of several competing stimuli. To elaborate further, attention is the process by which neural mechanisms assess and process this competition in order to create a unitary response (Desimone & Duncan, 1995). A very specific definition of selective attention is provided by Neibur and Koch (1998), "selective attention assures that we do not perceive a superposition of all stimuli present at a given time in our visual field, by suppressing the non-attended stimuli such that only one stimulus is processed at a given time in higher cortical areas" (p. 166). However, the term *focused attention* is sometimes used synonymously with *selective attention*, although processing is not always limited to one stimulus (Robbins, 1998). Arguably, research appears to be directed by these culturally created attention subcategories and not by neuroanatomy itself. All of these different subcategories, and their many definitions, create a fractured and unclear picture of attention as a concept.

Attention is difficult to define, and yet it is a concept deeply embedded in the western cultural construct for learning and behavior. The difficulties in defining attention are intensified when the study of attention is brought to the level of neurobiology because there appears to be no direct relationship between terminology and anatomy. Therefore, I suggest that attention as conceptualized and referred to in human behavior, particularly in language and learning, is a creation of culture and that this attention does not map isomorphically onto the brain. Attention is not subserved by a dedicated neural substrate. It is a process involving diverse anatomy and functions.

This chapter demonstrates that attention is a process in which biological mechanisms interact when goal-directed behaviors and stimulus-driven responses converge into action. This interaction occurs in moments so brief that we are not conscious of them as single units. Therefore, I characterize attention as a series of moments that make up a continuous process of evaluation, action, and reaction that is ever present in human behavior. The primary neurobiological participants in the attentional process are intrinsic properties of neurons, the dorsolateral prefrontal cortex, parietal cortex, frontoparietal circuits, and the anterior cingulate. This process is an ongoing exchange between neurobiology and environment, and its functions are not described by our cultural notion of *paying attention.*

When attention is defined as a fluid process, the borders that separate such concepts as attention, perception, cognition, and action are revealed as purely psychological without independent representation in the brain. For example, attention surely is part of perception, and perception part of cognition, and so on. In language as well, these concepts are not mutually exclusive, and their meaning depends on context. I propose that the overlap present in our cultural and psychological notions of perception, cognition, action, and attention is a reflection of functional overlap among neurobiological processes. The following section demonstrates that attention, as it occurs in the brain, is a process of interaction between learner and environment that depends on competition between behavioral goals, internal and external stimuli, and temporal contexts.

INFLUENCES OF GOAL-DIRECTED BEHAVIOR AND STIMULUS-DRIVEN RESPONSE

Inattentional Blindness

During the visual phenomenon of inattentional blindness behavioral goals and visual stimuli are in direct competition for processing resources. During tasks that illustrate inattentional blindness, participants are asked to determine which arm of a cross is longer, the vertical arm or the horizontal arm. The participants fixate on the cross and then an unexpected stimulus is presented near the crux. When the participants respond to the task, they are immediately asked if they see anything other than the two lines of the cross. Many participants report seeing only the cross. This result demonstrates the influence of the attentional goal (in this case, "pay attention to line length") over the perception of the visual environment (the unexpected stimulus) (Kanwisher & Wojciulik, 2000).

The question that emerges from this task is whether visual cortex processes all environmental details and then attention extracts specifics of a particular stimulus selected by behavioral goals, or whether attention restricts visual processing to only those goal specified stimulus details in the environment. Historically, according to Kanwisher and Wojciulik (2000), event related potential (ERP) research shows that behavioral goals affect stimulus processing in secondary visual cortices (extrastriate cortex [V2]), indicating that initial stimulus processing in primary visual cortex (V1) is not affected by the behavioral goals that influence attention. However, functional magnetic resonance imaging (fMRI) has repeatedly shown that behavioral goals modulate stimulus processing even in primary visual cortices (V1) (Kanwisher and Wojciulik, 2000; Martinez et al., 1999). These ERP and fMRI results may not be in conflict. Activity detected in V1 by the fMRI (a technology that gives high *spatial* resolution but poor temporal resolution) could reflect feedback from other areas of the brain (Martinez et al., 1999), whereas ERP results, which give a high *temporal* resolution, demonstrate the initial response to the stimulus, before feedback (Martinez et al., 1999). I hypothesize that behavioral goal information is transmitted to V1 by a feedback network before the entire processing of the stimulus is complete. This accounts for the conflicting fMRI and ERP results.

I propose that the combined spatial and temporal results indicate ongoing processing of the environment in which stimulus details are constantly being updated by input from behavioral goals, memory, motor plans, and homeostatic needs. In this scenario, when primary visual cortex (V1), and sec-

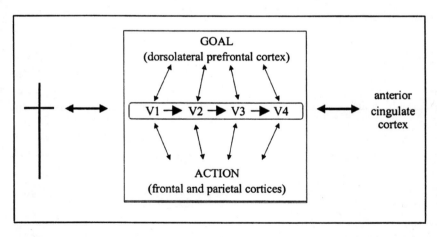

FIG. 6.1. Processing of a visual stimulus. Environmental stimulus details are detected by primary visual cortex (V1). This initial information is sent to secondary visual cortex (V2) as well as cortices involved in implementing goals and actions. These cortical areas send updated information back to V1 where it influences the detection of new environmental details and the ongoing processing of the original stimulus. V1 continues to send information to V2 and frontal and parietal cortices. This process of modulation and adjustment of stimulus information occurs at each stage of visual processing (V1, V2, V3, V4) creating a constant cycle of stimulus detection, refinement and redefinition according to goals and plans for action. Throughout the cycle the anterior cingulate cortex weighs the influences of goals and stimuli ensuring that the strongest influences are represented in an organism's response.

ondary visual cortex (V2), and so on (V3, V4) receive feedback, the processing of the stimulus is refined. Figure 6.1 (processing of a visual stimulus), demonstrates this refinement.

In the proposed operation, the initial environmental stimulus details are received by V1. Immediately V1 sends this information to V2 and to frontal and parietal areas involved in memory, goal formation and maintenance, and motor action, and to the anterior cingulate cortex, an area involved in coordinating internal and external influences on stimulus processing and response. Thus, initially, very general information from initial visual processing in V1 is sent to frontal and parietal cortices, and to the anterior cingulate cortex. This initial stimulus information is processed in these cortical areas and information is sent back to V1, creating a feedback network. This process takes place even before full recognition and processing of the stimulus has occurred. Additionally, stimulus information that has been only slightly more refined in V2 is being relayed to the same frontal and parietal cortices, anterior cingulate cortex, and feedback network. This same pattern would occur for the next stages of stimulus processing in V3 and V4. Area V1 continues to receive environmental input and, now the feedback as well (the same for V2, V3, etc.). Thus, a complex process that is cyclical in nature is created. In this hypothetical operation of stimulus perception and selection, information is sent to a feedback network at every step of processing. The influences of each of these steps are weighed by the anterior cingulate to determine priorities in the process of selecting and responding to a stimulus. This example shows the continuous nature of processing and negotiating the environment. In the context represented by Fig. 6.1, it is difficult to pinpoint the location or moment of attention.

After reviewing the visual processing of a simple stimulus, it is clear that attention should be approached as an interactive, temporal concept. In this context each moment in the process of attention is unique. For example, if the environment and stimulus has not changed and a stimulus is seen again, the temporal context of that perception has changed (i.e., feedback has affected the initial perception of the stimulus in V1). Furthermore, even if the behavioral goal remains the same, the stimulus environment may be altered. For example, in the inattentional blindness task (choosing the longer arm of a cross), a small, unexpected stimulus may go unnoticed. However, an unexpected, large, flashing star imposed on the same picture of the cross is likely to override the participant's task-specific goals because neurons in the visual pathway are innately receptive to stimulus properties such as novelty, color and incongruence (Desimone & Duncan, 1995; see section 3). Thus the length of the cross' arms may not even be detected. In this scenario, the unexpected qualities of color and movement in the stimulus compete for processing resources with the participant's goal.

The fMRI and ERP data discussed previously and the process represented by Fig. 6.1 suggest that within the processing of a single stimulus, behavioral goals and stimulus details prompt constant modulation and adjustment by way of a feedback network. This modulation occurs in several locations and times in the brain. If processing of a visual stimulus involves stimulus-driven response, goal-directed behavior, memory, and motor planning, then it appears that attention is all these things put together.

Covert Attention

Inattentional blindness demonstrates the interaction between stimuli and a simple task, based on a behavioral goal. Covert attention, where an object in the visual field may be noticed without physically orienting towards it, represents a more complex stimulus/goal interaction because there is no specific eye focus on new stimuli. An example of a covert attentional shift (as opposed to an overt attentional shift (OAS) in which a subject focuses on a new stimulus by moving the head or eye) can be demonstrated by the occulomotor delayed response (ODR) task in Fig. 6.2.

In this task, the eyes are focused on the target in the center location. The subject is trained to look at the center point for a 1 to 5 second period without any new foveation. During this period, a brief cue, such as the flash of a diamond, is presented in one of the outerlying squares. After a delay period, the center point stimulus is turned off and the subject, who has previously been instructed to do so, voluntarily orients (i.e., moves eye muscles in an action called a *saccade* or *foveation*) to the square in which he or she expects the next stimulus to appear. (The participant has been told the stimulus could appear in any square). Invariably, the subjects orient to the box in which the brief cue flashed. This task provides evidence that subjects' shift attention to, or notice, the cue, despite an absence of saccadic movement. This "noticing" is referred to as the Covert Attentional Shift (CAS).

Dorsolateral prefrontal cortex (DLPFC) activations that occur during CAS suggest that neurons are primed to maintain behavioral goals and/or working memory (Constantinidis, Williams, & Goldman-Rakic, 2002; Funehashi, Bruce, & Goldman-Rakic, 1990; Johnson, 1998). In monkeys performing the ODR task, during the period after the cue, and before the overt saccade, 80% of the neurons remaining active in the frontal eye field

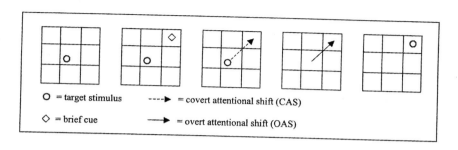

FIG. 6.2. Occulomotor Delayed Response (ODR) task. The target is initially located in the center square. The subject is trained to focus on the target for a 1 to 5 second period. During this time, a brief cue is given. The subject covertly "notices" the cue (CAS) while the eyes continue to focus on the target. Then, after a delay, the center target is removed and the subject refocuses (OAS) on a square where he or she most expects a new stimulus. Invariably this is the location where the cue appeared.

(FEF) and frontal sulcus (a possible homologue to the human DLPFC, Rushworth, Paus, & Sipila, 2001) were neurons that coded for the direction of the cue and future eye movements in that receptive field (Funehashi et al., 1990). This suggests that neurons are primed for expected action. This notion is supported by research into working memory that shows the inhibition of stimulus specific neurons unfolds over time linking stimulus representations (Constantinidis, et al. 2002).

The ODR task was adapted for infants (Gilmore & Johnson, 1995). Infants under 6 months of age could not delay the saccade to the location of the brief cue. In contrast, infants 6 months and older showed delayed overt attentional shifts, demonstrating results similar to those of monkeys (Johnson, 1998). These outcomes suggest that in the developing human brain, the DLPFC influences occulomotor control and attentional shift as early as 6 months of age. This research further indicates that whereas the subject focuses on the target in the center location for the trained 1 to 5 second period, another location is being held in memory by activated frontal neurons. It may be that this activation in frontal neurons is sustained; and then converted into motor action during the overt attentional shift. The ODR task highlights the necessary connections between the DLPFC, memory, and spatial and motor responses that involve parietal cortex. This research serves not only to define the phenomenon of CAS, but also demonstrates the development of early connections between frontal and parietal cortices and the central role these connections have in the attention process.

BIASED COMPETITION

Competition for Resources

Inattentional blindness and covert attention both illustrate the interplay and competition between the various elements of behavioral goals and environmental stimuli. The neurobiological details of this interplay and competition is explored further with an account of attention in object recognition as explained by biased competition. In general, object recognition is processed in what is called the *ventral stream* commonly called the *what pathway* (posterior parietal areas, to inferior temporal lobe, to ventral frontal lobe). The *dorsal stream*, commonly referred to as the *where pathway*, processes general spatial location (posterior parietal areas, to dorsal parietal cortex, to dorsal frontal lobe) (Webster & Ungerleider, 1998). There are three influences that define the process of object recognition: systems of chemical neurotransmitters, innate properties of neurons, and competition for resources. Object recognition is, in part, achieved through multiple levels of processing between sensory input and motor output and is likely to be mediated by systems of chemical neurotransmitters at all levels (Desimone & Duncan, 1995; Driver & Baylis, 1998; Robbins, 1998). Research on monkeys shows that the progression of object processing moves from primary visual areas through inferior posterior cortex, to temporal cortex, and finally, to the inferior temporal lobe (V1→V4→TEO→TE). See Fig. 6.3.

Following is a summary of object visual processing as described by Desimone and Duncan (1995). Neurons in each of the areas, V1, V4, TEO, and TE, have receptive fields that respond to stimuli in a specified area of the eye's visual field. V1 has the smallest receptive field at .2° and, thus, the most localized spatial temporal filter. For example, neurons in this area may respond only to movement of lines in a particular direction across a very small portion of the visual field. The V4 neuron receptive fields are measured at 3°, and TEO fields at 6°. As the neuronal fields become larger, they respond to broader defining qualities of an object, such as color, or curves versus angles. The inferior temporal (TE) neuronal receptive fields are very large, 25°, indicating that they respond to stimuli in a very large portion of the visual field. In

Monkey Brain

Human Brain

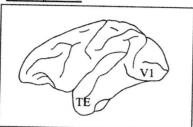
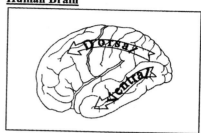

FIG. 6.3. Monkey brain and human brain. This representation of a monkey brain shows the first and last locations of visual object recognition as the primary visual cortex (V1) and the monkey inferior temporal lobe (TE). In the figure of the human brain, object recognition is represented by the "what" pathway, also called the *ventral stream*, whereas spatial location is represented by the "where" pathway, known as the *dorsal stream*.

contrast to V1 cells, TE cells can select for much larger spatial definitions such as an entire shape.

When multiple objects are in the visual field, properties of these objects are processed by overlapping receptive fields. The properties that elicit the most response from trait-specific receptive fields are likely to have greater neural representation (Desimone & Duncan, 1995; O'Scalaidhe, Wilson, & Goldman-Rakic, 1999). This leads to competition among objects for processing resources (i.e., representation and recognition by cells' receptive fields). This competition may account for the slower target (environmental stimulus) selection times and higher error rates found in divided attention tasks, where the subject has to choose among multiple, similar targets (Braun, 1998; Desimone & Duncan, 1995). The posterior and dorsal parietal cortex (homologues to *TEO/IT* in the ventral stream) also have neurons with increasingly larger and larger receptive fields, indicating that selection of a target stimulus, by means of competition for resources, occurs in the dorsal stream as well (Desimone & Duncan, 1995). With competitive selection active in both the ventral and dorsal streams, there must be a mechanism that ensures that these processing streams select the same objects. This mechanism could be working memory, an attentional template, the anterior cingulate, systems of chemical neurotransmitters, or a process that relies on all of these, such as attention.

Innate Neural Response to External Stimuli

There are two general forms of influence on target selection: stimulus-driven influences generated by the environment, and goal-directed influences generated from within the organism (i.e., memory, existing motor plans, homeostatic needs, general behavioral and task-related goals; Desimone & Duncan, 1995; Driver & Frith, 2000; Fadiga, Fogassi, Gallese, & Rizzolatti, 1998; Iacoboni, 2000; Milner, 1999; Posner & DiGirolamo, 1998; Robbins, 1998). These influences are components of the attention process and create biases that guide an organism's actions. As we have seen in tasks that reveal inattentional blindness, some physical properties of a stimulus elicit pre-programmed neural activation and thereby a bias is formed that overrides the task goal. For example, a novel or incongruent stimulus, such as the flashing red star, or one that is larger or redder than others in the visual field, is likely to create a bias for its own selection by commanding more response from neuronal receptive fields in multiple levels of the ventral stream.

One form of stimulus-driven bias is formed by a nonhomogeneous object within a homogeneous background, such as a red square amid yellow circles. This is called the *pop-out effect*. The anatomy of the visual system is designed to detect novelties and abnormalities in the visual field that pop-out (Braun, 1998; Nakayama & Joseph, 1998). In contrast, in "divided attention," the task goal requires searching for a target with specific features that distinguish it from other similar stimuli. This involves greater competition and can take more time and/or produce higher rates of error (Braun, 1998). For example, in a group of circles, where the target circle size is just slightly smaller than the others but all other features are shared, the distinguishing feature is a slight difference in size and it does not pop-out, thus the target is harder to identify. Figure 6.4 illustrates the effects of divided attention. The pop out effect is an example of a strong stimulus driven/intrinsic bias, whereas divided attention demonstrates more clearly the competition between task goal and environmental stimuli.

The internal, behavioral bias is made up of the properties of a goal that affect stimulus processing as well. For example, the organism's goal may be to "find the red square" or to "ignore the red square." In this manner, internal influences that create bias are still dependent on the physical qualities of a stimulus but involve memory and an organism's intention, or action plan, as well. These internal biases could be implemented by an attentional template, working memory or short-term memory, or frontoparietal circuits, all of which are further discussed in section 4 (Awh & Jonides, 1998; Corbetta, 1998; Desimone & Duncan, 1995; Fuster, 1995).

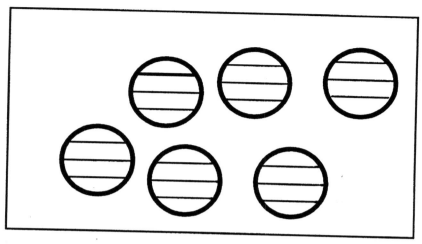

FIG. 6.4. Circles with shared features. These circles share several characteristics: shape, stripes, color, and line thickness. The distinguishing feature of the target stimulus is line thickness of the top-most stripe. The stripe is thicker than the others. This feature is in minimal contrast to the others, thus it is comparatively more difficult to detect. This effect is called *divided attention*.

Internal Stimuli

The attention process involves several aspects of memory or experience, which I label internal stimuli. Internal stimuli affect target stimulus selection. These stimuli can be novel and familiar, and from recent experience, all of which are defined by temporal context. Novel items in the visual field may invoke an automatic neural response and thus bias competition in their favor (Desimone & Duncan, 1995; Nakayama & Joseph, 1998). However, familiarity with a stimulus produces strong competition for resources as well, possibly due to stored information in memory and/or neural circuitry (Corbetta, 1998; Nakayama & Joseph, 1998). The Fig. 6.5 represents a task that involves familiar stimuli and an unexpected or 'novel' presentation of those stimuli. In this task, the time required to find the inverted numeral target is independent of the number of upright numerals (Braun, 1998; Desimone & Duncan, 1995). This suggests that it is the unfamiliar, novel visual presentation (the inverted numeral) that pops out and is noticed.

An example of a familiarity bias is when one hears a familiar name called in a crowd of noisy people. One hears that name rather than all the other words

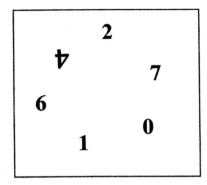 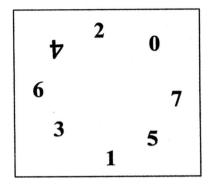

FIG. 6.5. Inverted numerals. The upside down number "stands out" among the others because of its unusual presentation. Unlike divided attention, it does not matter how many right side up numbers are in the display, the target stimulus is sufficiently different from the other stimuli and it is easy to find. This is called the *pop-out effect*.

spoken. In this case, the name is noticed as a stimulus incongruent with its background. Additionally, a familiar stimulus can counteract the influence of a novel stimulus. For example, a subject produces more errors when trying to select a novel target if overlearned visual targets are also present (Braun, 1998; Corbetta, 1998; Iacoboni, 2000). Essentially, the subject notices the familiar target first due to an internal stimulus bias from memory. This has been shown with studies of occulomotor behavior and attentional shifts in which stimulus induced saccadic eye movement is influenced by the location of previous saccades (Corbetta, 1998). These dual effects of novelty and familiarity may be significant in language learning and will be discussed in the section, "Attention in Adult Second Language Learning."

An additional influence on selection, often working in tandem with familiarity, is recency (Corbetta, 1998; Nakayama et al., 1998). The most recently seen stimuli produce a smaller neural signal in the visual cortex when the same stimuli are presented a second time (Corbetta, 1998). These results seem to indicate that neurons that would initially respond to general features of a stimulus, such as direction of movement, do not fire the second time around. Instead, only those neurons that respond to both general and specific stimulus features would activate. This suggests that recently seen stimuli may evoke stored activation patterns represented as "primed" neurons (Desimone & Duncan, 1995; Nakayama et al., 1998). One could imagine that this record of previous stimuli could be due to cortical storage or memory formation involving frontoparietal circuitry, cortex, hippocampus, basal ganglia, and other structures. Priming and inhibition may be how memories (i.e., activations prompted by stimulus properties) are retained from trial to trial (Johnson, 1998). The details of memory formation, although intricately woven with the attention process, are beyond the present scope of this chapter (see chaps. 3-5, this volume).

Memory or experience can cause inhibition of neuron activation and thus affect novel target stimulus selection (Desimone & Duncan, 1995; Miller, 2000). This indicates that, as one learns the distinguishing features of the stimulus, the neuron receptive fields that activate to general stimulus properties stop responding to the stimulus, and only those predesigned for the features unique to the target stimulus are activated (Desimone & Duncan, 1995). In this case, overall selectivity may be increased while inhibition causes the actual quantity of neuronal activation to decrease (O'Scalaidhe et al., 1999).

In summary, three aspects of memory or experience, novelty, familiarity, and recency all influence visual selective attention via mechanisms such as priming or inhibition. Cells that are selective for a goal- determined target are primed prior to the presentation of the target stimulus (Desimone & Duncan, 1995; Fadiga, Fogassi, Gallese, & Rizzolatti, 2000; Iacoboni, 2000; Miller, 2000). According to biased competition, this priming would result in competition between the primed cells and those that are most responsive to the stimulus properties of novelty, and, familiarity, and recency. Priming is likely a result of a target selection guide or memory biased by behavioral goals. Studies in working memory point to the prefrontal cortex as a source for attentional goals (Awh & Jonides 1998; Corbetta, 1998).

THE ATTENTIONAL GOAL

The DLPFC and Working Memory

In terms of visual processing, an attentional goal could be very limited as in the task goal, "search for the color red," or it could involve a search for several object features such as color, shape, and movement. The visual system interacts with, or is influenced by, internal states such as memory and emotion, resulting in visual "awareness," possibly another term for "noticing." These internal states contribute to a behavioral goal sometimes labeled, the *attentional bias* (Corbetta, 1998). Corbetta proposed that these states are at least partially represented in source signals (representing object and feature, or location) that originate in the right prefrontal cortex, the same areas involved in working memory tasks.

As previously discussed, memory and attention and their subcategories are not entirely separate entities. There are similarities in descriptive terminology and shared neurobiological functions for both memory and attention. The right prefrontal cortex frequently shows activity during tasks requiring working memory (Awh & Jonides, 1998; Corbetta, 1998; de Fockert, 2001; Fuster, 1996). Working memory may be a part of, or synonymous with, the attentional goal. For example, locational working memory has been found in the superior frontal region near premotor, Brodmann's area 6 (Awh & Jonides, 1998; Corbetta, 1998). This area projects to, and employs, the superior parietal region (Brodmann's area 40) to coordinate spatial and nonspatial visual processing, which involves attention (Awh & Jonides, 1998). However, when attention to multiple feature detection is necessary, the right middle prefrontal region, near Brodmann's area 45/46, is involved in object oriented working memory (Corbetta, 1998). It is possible that the qualities of environmental stimuli require processing unique to these areas. If this is the case, then the regions previously mentioned (Brodmann's area 6, Brodmann's area 45/46) would not correspond to a type of memory or subcategory of attention but rather would be responsive to specific stimulus qualities. For example, object grasping and preparation for grasping activate Brodmann's area 45. Thus, when object detection is part of a task-goal, then working memory would appear object oriented and employ Brodmann's area 45 among other regions.

Another subcategory of memory that is intertwined with task goals, and thus, the attentional process, is *active short term memory* (Fuster, 1996). Fuster found that active short term memory engages regions (Brodmann's area 45/46), described as the DLPFC, during nonspatial matching tasks. The DLPFC appears to be involved in many subcategories of memory. In addition, it is activated during a variety of attention tasks (de Fockert et al., 2001; MacDonald, Cohen, Stenger, & Carter, 2000; Milham et al., 2001). However, like the working memory research reviewed above, the literature on the DLPFC and attention describes a variety of roles, definitions, and levels of involvement. MacDonald et al. (2000) found a general role for the DLPFC, concluding that it maintains and represents attentional demands of a task. However, de Fockert et al. (2001) suggested that working memory controls selective attention because the prefrontal cortex shows increased activation during divided attention tasks in which target selection accuracy is reduced in the presence of several distracting stimuli. This indicates that increased memory load affects the attention process (de Fockert et al., 2001).

Milham et al. (2001) defined the attentional role of the frontal cortex with greater detail, delineating distinct DLPFC functions for the right and left hemispheres. Using time delayed stroop tasks, they found activation in several regions within the right hemisphere: inferior frontal gyrus (Brodmann's area 44), middle frontal gyrus (Brodmann's area 9), superior frontal gyrus (Brodmann's areas 8/9), and superior parietal lobule (Brodmann's area 7). These areas were activated only during tasks that involved incongruent or competing possible responses. These results suggest that the right hemisphere plays a role in attentional control at action or response stages. In contrast, activation of left hemisphere regions, middle frontal gyrus (Brodmann's area 9/6), precuneus cortex (Brodmann's area 7), and superior parietal lobe (Brodmann's area 7) was significant during preresponse stages of the same tasks involving incongruent responses. These findings may indicate a left hemisphere role in attention when conflict arises during establishing and maintaining sensory representation and task goals. Activation in the parietal and frontal cortices of both hemispheres suggests a complex interplay between frontal and parietal cortices in selective attention tasks (Awh & Jonides, 1998; Corbetta, 1998; Fuster, 1996; Milham et al., 2001). These circuits, however, may not be specific to attention. For example, Fuster interprets the high degree of connections between frontal and parietal areas as the basic component of spatial working memory (1996).

This research demonstrates the complexity and intertwined nature of working memory, goals, and attention. The functional overlap and neuroanatomy shared by working memory and attention is illustrated in Table 6.1. The DLPFC is activated in all six of the studies listed, regardless of whether the authors are studying short-term memory, working memory, attentional control, or attentional demands.

It appears that aspects of memory and attention are the same process. In fact, neuroanatomical activations shared by spatial working memory and spatial selective attention may directly reflect shared functions (Awh & Jonides, 1998). From this perspective, an attentional template could simply be a task goal, held in memory, that contributes to stimulus selection and response. This view of attention allows the hypothesis that the attention process used in the broad category of language learning is similar to visual attention except that it would involve a wider range of cortical areas, such as auditory processing, tactile processing, and so on (Duncan & Owen, 2000).

TABLE 6.1

Working Memory and Attention Tasks Employ the Cortical Regions

DLPFC-Parietal	Spatial working memory/spatial selective attention	Awh & Jonides, 1998
DLPFC	Working memory/attentional bias	Corbetta, 1998
PFC	Working memory controls visual selective attention	De Fockert et al., 2001
DLPFC	Active short term memory	Fuster, 1996
DLPFC-Parietal	Spatial working memory	Fuster, 1996
DLPFC	Maintains and represents attentional demands	MacDonald et al., 2000
Rt. DLPFC-Parietal	Attentional control for action, response	Milham et al., 2001
Left DLPFC-Parietal	Attentional control for stimulus representation, behavioral goal	Milham et al., 2001

Motor Attention

Attention, as it functions in learning, cannot be fully understood without addressing the behavioral goal, also referred to as *intention*. Extracting intention from attention is analogous to separating memory from attention, because they rely on the same neural structures. However, Rushworth, Krams, and Passingham (2001a) suggested that there exists a clear, anatomical distinction between visuospatial perception, which they label "attention," and motor planning, which they refer to as *intention*, or *motor attention*. They claimed this distinction is represented most clearly in parietal lobe anatomy of both macaques and humans. In a separate paper, Rushworth, Paus, and Sipila (2001b) proposed that the human posterior intraparietal sulcus is specific to visuospatial orienting. In the macaque, the posterior inferior parietal gyrus (7a) and the adjacent posterior lateral intraparietal area (LIP) are thought to be specific to visuospatial orienting (Rushworth et al., 2001b). Areas 7a and LIP receive input from dorsal visual areas and project to the frontal eye fields (FEF). The dominant neurons in these areas are visually responsive neurons. Rushworth et al. (2001b) suggested that the right human posterior intraparietal sulcus is homologous to 7a and LIP of the macaque, and, thus, also specific to visuospatial orienting. In contrast, in humans, the left anterior intraparietal sulcus and supramarginal gyrus showed significant activation for motor attention during PET tasks that involved limb movement. Rushworth et al. (2001a) hypothesized that the distinct trajectories of the sylvian fissure in the two human hemispheres may allow for a larger supramarginal gyrus in the left anterior parietal lobe and increased posterior parietal areas near the angular gyrus in the right hemisphere. These distinctions would account for the right lateralization for orienting and the left lateralization for motor attention. The anterior intraparietal sulcus and supramarginal gyrus of the left hemisphere are likely homologues to the anterior inferior parietal area (7b) and the adjacent anterior intraparietal area (AIP) of the macaque (Rushworth et al., 2001b). In the macaque, areas 7b and AIP contain a mix of visual and motor neurons that respond both to somatosensation and limb movement. These areas receive somatosensory input and project to the ventral premotor area. The ventral premotor region of the macaque may have a homologue in the human inferior precentral sulcus region. Rushworth et al. (2001b) found that, in human imaging studies, the inferior precentral sulcus region activated during motor attention, indicating a frontoparietal circuit for motor attention or intention.

To Rushworth et al. (2001a), these correlations between the macaque brain and the human brain suggest that the left hemisphere supramarginal gyrus and anterior intraparietal sulcus are specific to a motor attention that is activated in response to visual and/or somatic stimuli that elicit motor response and thus the intention to act. However, it can be argued that *all* attentive behavior is motor and involves preparation of motor action in the form of saccades. In fact, research has repeatedly shown that participants in attentional tasks react faster if, while waiting for the stimulus, they covertly attend to the motor action they will make during a response rather than thinking about the expected visual stimulus (Iacoboni, 2000). Therefore, even initial processing of the expected stimulus is affected by motor planning. For example, if a participant is instructed to push a button when the expected stimulus appears in the visual field, the response is faster when the participant attends to pushing the button while still directing his or her visual focus on the visual field. If he or she simply looks at the visual field without any covert attention to action planning, in this "button-pushing" task, the response time is not as fast. Therefore, if action planning affects the perception of a stimulus and the interpretation of the environment, then the distinctions between stimulus perception and action response are blurry and divisions between perception, action, and intention appear purely semantic. In this light, separate attentional systems for perception and intention or response, like those proposed by Rushworth and colleagues, are implausible.

Visuospatial processing and motor planning are integrated parts of the attention process. Fadiga, Fogassi, Gallese, and Rizzolatti (2000) argued that eye movement, or oculomotor action, relates to spatial coordinate points that are specific to the body part (i.e., arm, leg, fingers) involved in acting on a particular stimulus. If this is the case, there is no specific visuospatial attention that selects stimuli. Instead, the properties of the stimulus itself and innate mechanisms for processing those properties, such as the size and specificity of neuronal receptive field, evoke cortical activations for actions like finger movement and preplanned saccades. Whether or not these plans are executed depends on input from behavioral goals, represented in working memory and internal stimuli such as declarative memory, and/or homeostasis. From this data, it appears that motor planning and particularly occulomotor planning (preplanned saccades) are necessary for the perception and interpretation of stimuli and therefore an essential element of the attention process.

Attention as Preparation for Action

Attention, and specifically covert attention, appear to always involve occulomotor planning or intentions for action (Corbetta, 1998; Corbetta & Schulman, 2002; Iacoboni, 2000). However, this notion is challenged by research presenting rapidly changing stimuli at the point of fixation, where presumably no new motor plan would need to be formed. During these tasks, motor areas of the intraparietal sulcus still show large activations that increase in proportion to the number of attended stimuli (Kanwisher & Wojciulik, 2000). Kanwisher and Wojciulik argued that because there is no need for occulomotor planning in this task, the intraparietal and frontal activations in visual attention tasks do not represent preplanned saccades. They use these results to argue for the existence of a "pure" attention, as yet undefined, which employs both parietal and frontal areas, and does not involve occulomotor planning.

It can be argued however, that although motor planning appears to be unnecessary in the previously mentioned task, it might improve performance. For example, the preparation for grasping an object improves the *detection* of visual stimuli that share essential properties with the target to be grasped (Fadiga et al., 2000). In essence, motor planning is in effect before the processing of a stimulus is complete, such that the anticipation of an action response actually assists and shapes the processing of a stimulus. If this is so, then activity in the intraparietal sulcus, like that detected by Kanwisher and Wojciulik, could represent part of a motor planning circuit activated by grasping preparation. One could speculate that this planning would enhance the processing of a repeated visual stimulus by refining the processing of the distinct stimulus quality and inhibiting activation of unneeded neuronal receptive fields (see section, "Internal Stimuli"). Thus, even a pure attention such as that proposed by Kanwisher and Wojciulik (2000) would include motor planning that would activate both frontal cortex (premotor cortex, presupplementary motor area, DLPFC) and parietal cortex (IPA, secondary visual processing areas). Furthermore, a specific type of attention, such as a "motor attention," like that supported by Rushworth et al. (2001a, b), may just be a label for a part of the process of attention in which stimulus-driven response and goal-directed behavior elicit limb movement, which in turn, activates the intraparietal area.

Frontoparietal Networks

Another possible scenario that could account for the parietal activations found by Kanwisher and Wojciulik in the repeated visual stimulus tasks is that the frontal and parietal activations noted by Kanwisher and Wojciulik are an indication of frontoparietal circuits that activate with attentive behavior. Even if visual stimulus tasks do not evoke oculomotor planning, "intention," or "plans for action," it may be that the parietal and frontal activations are not part of a pure attention, but were evoked solely by the properties of the external stimulus itself, or by reactivation of internal stimuli, such as goals and memory. Frontoparietal networks are implicated in both working memory (Awh & Jonides, 1998; Fuster, 1996) and visual attentional behavior (Corbetta 1998; Corbetta & Schulman, 2002; Milham et al., 2001). Additionally, attentional behavior in other modalities, as well as in mathematical abilities and general intelligence relies, in part, on frontoparietal networks (Duncan & Owen, 2000; Kanwisher & Wojciulik, 2000; Miller, 2000).

Based on human fMRI data, Corbetta and Schulman (2002) outlined a dorsal frontoparietal network subserving goal-directed sensory selection and response in both hemispheres. Specifically, this network includes cortex indicated in many types of attention research (Milham et al., 2001; Rushworth et al., 2001a, b). The network consists of the dorsal frontal cortex (at the intersection of the precentral and superior sulci) and the intraparietal sulcus, which are thought to be homologues to the frontal eye fields (FEF) and the lateral intraparietal region (LIP) of the monkey, respectively. Both these areas were found to be involved in anticipating activity before a stimulus and in planning for hand and eye movement. In monkeys, the LIP and FEF show activation for four types of tasks—those involving attention, working memory, eye movement, or expectation of a stimulus (Corbetta & Shulman, 2002; Kanwisher & Wojciulik, 2000). Corbetta and Schulman argued that all of these tasks are involved in the assembly and coordination of response to a stimulus.

Summary of the "Attentional Goal"

It has been demonstrated that there is little distinction between working memory and the attentional goals that activate the DLPFC. Additionally, the possibility of a motor attention, based in the intraparietal sulcus, was explored. I argue that there is no specific motor attention and that all attentive behavior involves preplanned saccades, and may involve other preplanned motor activity. The fact that some of this planning may even enhance the processing of a visual stimulus highlights the interactive nature of the attentional process. Furthermore, several authors suggested that connections between frontal areas and parietal cortex play a key role in action planning and stimulus response (Corbetta et al., 2002; Milham et. al., 2000; Rushworth et al., 2001a). I propose that these frontoparietal circuits provide the additional feedback necessary to constantly update the processing of a visual stimulus. This is illustrated in Fig. 6.6 shown here. This figure is a revised version of Fig. 6.1 (processing of a visual stimu-

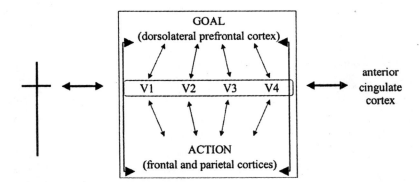

FIG. 6.6. Processing of a visual stimulus-revised. Environmental stimulus details are detected by primary visual cortex (V1). This initial information is sent to secondary visual cortex (V2) as well as the frontal and parietal cortices that are involved in implementing goals and actions. Frontal and parietal connections further enhance the stimulus processing. These cortical areas send updated information back to V1 where it influences the detection of new environmental details and the ongoing processing of the original stimulus. V1 continues to send information to V2 and frontal and parietal cortices. This process of modulation and adjustment of stimulus information occurs at each stage of visual processing (V1, V2, V3, V4) creating a constant cycle of stimulus detection, refinement, and redefinition according to goals and plans for action. Throughout the cycle the anterior cingulate cortex weighs the influences of goals and stimuli ensuring that the strongest influences are represented in an organism's response.

lus), which represents the influences of frontoparietal circuits over stimulus selection and response.

Detection/Response as One Action

Frontoparietal circuits are a candidate for the component of the attention process that blends target selection and target response. According to Fadiga et al. (2000), frontal areas, such as Brodmann's area 6, show several distinct divisions with bidirectional parallel circuits connecting the frontal and parietal cortices. This indicates a multilevel integration of functions and communication between sensory input and associations in the parietal cortex, and motor output based in the frontal cortex (Fadiga et al., 2000). Bidirectional circuits would facilitate the flow of information regarding the refinement of stimulus processing. Mirror neurons provide further evidence for frontoparietal circuits that contribute to stimulus processing and, ultimately, attentive behavior. Frontal areas of the monkey brain, FEF, F4, and F5, are the regions most heavily projected to from the inferior parietal lobe. In these areas are ventral premotor neurons, commonly referred to as *mirror neurons*, which have a dual response pattern (Fadiga et al., 2000). They fire in response to sensory tactile stimuli prompting motor action, as well as in response to visual stimuli, or perception. According to Fadiga et al. (2000), the dual nature of F4 neurons reflects the presence of potential action plans, or motor schemata, evoked by a visual stimulus. As reviewed earlier in "Motor Attention," preparing for a grasping action enhances the processing of a visual stimulus with traits that match those of the object to be grasped (Fadiga et al., 2000). These preparations may or may not be carried out depending on behavioral goals affecting varying levels of processing. This indicates that a subject's motor interaction with the environment contributes to the organisms processing of sensory events such that a motor response affects the target stimulus selected for and the way that the stimulus processing is refined.

In this process biases created by behavioral goals and motor preparation enhance an organism's interpretation of the environment and thus affect the processing of the stimulus. In short, 'expectation' influences stimulus selection and interpretation (Driver & Frith, 2000). One element of this picture, the anterior cingulate cortex, has not been discussed. In this hypothetical process, I propose that the anterior cingulate cortex acts as a competitive weigh station assessing influences from possible responses and sending feedback to cerebral cortex.

THE ANTERIOR CINGULATE AND THE ATTENTION NETWORK

The details regarding the relationship between working memory, the DLPFC, parietal areas and attention or attentional tasks are still a matter of some debate. However, there is considerable agreement that the anterior cingulate cortex assists in bringing together behavioral goals, plans for action, and influences from external and internal stimuli (Botvinick, Nystrom, Fissell, Carter, & Cohen, 1999; Carter et al., 1998; Corbetta, 1998; MacDonald et al., 2000; Milham et al., 2001). The anterior cingulate is a midline structure considered limbic in nature. However, the curved and distributed anatomical form of the cingulate ensures its contact with diverse neuroanatomy such as premotor areas (for instance, the pre-supplementary motor area (pre-SMA)), the amygdala, considered an area critically involved in emotion, and the hippocampus, associated with declarative memory formation (see chap. 4, this volume). Due to this central location and high level of connections to various anatomy, the anterior cingulate is considered essential to attention and decision making processes (Botvinick et al., 1999; Carter et al., 1998; Corbetta, 1998; MacDonald et al. 2000; Milham et al. 2001).

In classic attention models, the anterior cingulate is characterized as a funnel for frontal lobe generated biases being sent to posterior visual processing regions (LaBerge, 1995; Marrocco & Davidson, 1998; Posner, 1990, 1994, 1998). Classic attention research has also suggested that the anterior cingulate performs the role of error-detector during processing (Corbetta, 1998; Posner & Dahaene, 1994; Posner & DiGirolamo, 1998; Posner & Petersen, 1990). Many imaging studies show significant anterior cingulate activity when a selection mistake is made during an attentional task. Therefore, it is often concluded that the anterior cingulate activity is in response to, or prompted by, the selection error (Posner & DiGirolamo, 1998; Corbetta, 1998). However, the anterior cingulate is often activated even during tasks associated with low error rates, such as the Stroop task, and tasks measuring verbal fluency (Carter et al., 1998). The anterior cingulate also shows activation during correct target selection responses (Carter et al., 1998; Posner & DiGirolamo, 1998). Given the anterior cingulate activation in both correct and incorrect responses, Carter et al. (1998) argued that the anterior cingulate performs a comparator function that monitors competition between conflicting aspects of the attention process.

Carter et al. proposed that the anterior cingulate uses inhibitory mechanisms to weigh competing inputs from frontal, parietal, and midbrain areas, in a process similar to biased competition at the neuronal level (Carter et al., 1998). For example, it has been suggested that people with schizophrenia exhibit altered attentive behavior due to a loss of inhibitory function in the anterior cingulate cortex (Benes, 1993; Nestor & O'Donnell, 1998; Posner & DiGirolamo, 1998). In schizophrenic patients (who, in general, perform poorly on attention tasks) the cingulate has an increased number of glutamatergic (excitatory) inputs and a diminished number of inhibitory GABA inputs and receptors (Posner & DiGirolamo, 1998). Nestore and O'Donnell (1998) introduced the notion that disturbances of GABAergic inhibitory interneurons alone may account for schizophrenic attentional abnormalities. These abnormalities result in reduced regulatory neuronal firing in the cingulate. Without inhibitory firing, the anterior cingulate cortex may not be able to properly weigh the influences from working memory, behavioral goals, internal stimuli, and so on. Information from all of these sources may be relayed to cortical areas (such as V3, and V4, as seen in Fig. 6.6) involved in refining the detection and response to the stimulus, even if that information is conflicting. Thus, the attention process and behavior in general could be negatively affected, as is evident in the case of schizophrenia. Therefore it appears that, in a normal organism, the anterior cingulate is constantly inhibiting possible response or action plans that have inferior influence, or weight, such that the tonic inhibitory state of the anterior cingulate would provide necessary feedback for target selection/stimulus processing. Furthermore, this research suggests that the anterior cingulate acts as an inhibitory mechanism, constantly involved in all behavior requiring attention. The anterior cingulate is likely part of a network that maintains optimal performance and within this network it provides negative feedback (MacDonald et al., 2000).

As part of this network, the anterior cingulate is affected by temporal context. For example, Botvinivck et al. (1999) found that if initial trials involved high conflict, then anterior cingulate activation was greater in the subsequent trials. This indicates an interaction between trials that occurs when recently seen stimuli create an internal temporal environment for stimulus detection using the phenomenon of priming.

Anterior cingulate activation is affected by conflicting response plans, action execution, and internal and external stimuli that bias the processing of stimuli and response to stimuli. The research reviewed above suggests that the anterior cingulate is indeed part of a network that maintains optimal performance. However, it must be noted that any of these biases may lead to a response that is incorrect as well. For example, recency and familiarity ex-

ert great influence on response patterns, and may cause the organism to select the most recently seen stimulus, even if it is not selected for by the task
goal. In this situation, the anterior cingulate would be activated even in the
case of error. Further research regarding the anterior cingulate's role in the
network and other candidates for neurobiological mechanisms that help
maintain optimal performance has been restricted by the limitations of
fMRI technology (MacDonald et al., 2000). However, attention, as defined
in language and culture, certainly seems necessary for performance, as do
all the processes described here in attentional research. It may be that the
"network for optimal performance," to borrow MacDonald et al.'s term, is
the network for attention, and that maintenance of behavior and stimulus
detection/response is attention itself.

ATTENTION AS AN INTEGRATED NETWORK

Individual properties of neurons, high levels of frontal-parietal interconnectivity, and a meshing of sensory and motor functions, all create the phenomenon, so often referred to as attention. In light of this view, and the notion
of neural competition, the standard psychological concept of attention that
guides so much of attentional research loses its descriptive accuracy.
Frontoparietal connectivity supports a multilevel integrated view of an attention that depends on internal stimuli, external stimuli, and the temporal context. Milner (1999) and Iacoboni (2000) supported the notion that a unitary
conceptual label like attention is not applicable to the brain. An integrated view
of attention in which neurobiological processes and functions of the body
proper are central is a more accurate way of understanding attention and its role
in learning and behavior.

According to Iacoboni (2000), attention is not subserved by dedicated neural
substrates. Instead what is labeled attention is really an outcome of activity in
frontoparietal sensorimotor circuits (like those previously discussed by Fadiga et
al.) that results in stimuli selecting for a response, *and* responses selecting stimuli.
Iacoboni (2000) supported this assertion by citing PET and fMRI data showing
similar activation in these circuits during simple motor tasks such as finger tapping
and attentional tasks involving target selection. In this view of attention, and in
cognition more generally, a subject interacts with the environment and cognition
arises from that interaction. The subject is not limited to passive reception of stimuli but actually influences which stimuli are reacted to. Iacoboni (2000) went so far
as to suggest that the "boundaries between perception, cognition, and action are
fictitious" (p. 464).

Attention is an interactive process between the organism's overall behavioral goals, task goals, and current homeostatic needs, his or her internal stimuli, external stimuli, and the fluid temporal context. All of these elements converge to create attentional behavior. This behavior affects what we interact with and how we learn. For an adult second language learner, personal history, the language learning environment, and goals all become elements of the attention process.

ATTENTION IN SECOND LANGUAGE LEARNING

Attention in adult second language learning is a reflection of the interaction between learner and the learning environment, whether it is in a classroom or an immersion setting. In this section I hypothesize about the roles played by the various elements of attention in second language acquisition. A learner's temporal context, as defined by the environment and internal goals and memories, has great impact on language learning. In conversation, the interlocutor is often the most influential part of the environment, and his or her speech can have profound impact on what and how one talks and responds (Haiman, 1983).

The Temporal Context of the Learner

Attentive behavior in learning is influenced by the temporal context of the internal and external environment of the organism. The internal temporal context is composed of several items including language learning goals, daily and task-based goals, and a learner's personal history. Aspects of personal history, such as academic history, individual learning style, and preferences for methods of instruction each affect learning (Ellis, 1995; Skehan, 1998). A student's history of language learning success, and general homeostatic needs are also part of the temporal context. Schumann and Wood (this volume) discuss how a learner's motivation can affect SLA success. They tell the story of Barbara, who studied French in school but did not gain any real proficiency. However, approximately 10 years later when she had a French speaking boyfriend, Barbara again studied French and she excelled. Schumann and Wood hypothesize that this success was primarily due to a greater motivation, that is, the desire to communicate with her boyfriend. Partially because of her success with French, Barbara later went on to study both Spanish and German. However, when studying these languages, she did not have the same motivation she had when learning French, and she achieved only limited success (in Spanish and German). The story of Barbara demonstrates the role of motivation in learning and the impact one's history of language learning may or may not have on continued and future language learning for the individual. Thus, it is evident the temporal context, including personal history, success, and motivation affect attentional behavior and second language learning in the adult.

Visual Stimulus Processing as a Model for Second Language Processing

In visual processing, there are innate properties of neurons that respond to novel and incongruent stimuli. It is also true that recently seen stimuli and previous motor actions may cause priming that affects the processing of new stimuli (Corbetta, 1998; Fadiga et al., 2000; Iacaboni, 2000). There are indications that neurons function in a similar manner in cortices involved in other modalities, such as audition (Desimone & Duncan, 1995; Duncan & Owen, 2000; Kanwisher & Wojciulik, 2000; O'Scalaidhe et al. 1999). If one imagines that other areas of the brain involved in learning also have neurons that respond to memory, motor planning, novelty, and incongruity, then one can assume that salient linguistic input could elicit greater response than less salient stimuli, and thus create bias in the attention process.

External Stimuli

Like in the temporal context, stimuli in the learning environment affect attentional behavior. These stimuli may be processed in the same way visual stimuli are processed. For example, novel vocabulary words in the L2 may, pop-out, that is, elicit a general response from a greater number of neurons, than already learned vocabulary. However, it is also possible that the listener might not even notice this novel vocabulary because it would not be familiar, and thus there would be no internal stimulus from memory influencing processing resources.

Internal Stimuli

Novel and incongruent stimuli automatically evoke neural response. However, information stored in memory, acting as internal stimuli, could overpower the influences of novelty and incongruity. In visual processing, neurons that respond to recently processed stimuli are more likely to remain primed and to become active again, if subsequent stimuli are the same, or if they share qualities with those stimuli that primed the neurons. I propose that novel stimuli, priming, and recency have the same affect on second language learning. For example, if a student recently learned the grammatical rule " third person singular present tense takes the morpheme -s," that student may be more likely to *notice* this form in linguistic social interaction. This rule, held in declarative memory, could constitute priming. These primed neurons could then exert influence over initial processing of the external stimulus (the linguistic interaction), and, as the learner creates a response, contribute a strong bias to be weighed by the anterior cingulate.

Procedural knowledge is also an internal stimulus. It could affect the role of attention in learning by creating biases for grammatical rules, vocabulary sequences, or phrases, which a student may have over-learned. For instance, many adult second language learners continue to use variations of the simple present, such as "Jane walk to school every day," even when they are overtly taught or exposed to the correct grammatical use of third person singular "-s," "Jane walks to school." In these situations, it may be likely that an over-learned simple expression of time, "everyday," exerts a more powerful influence than the less practiced grammatical morpheme '-s.' Additionally, behavioral goals could stress the need to communicate over the need to use correct grammar. Hence, the learner uses available common vocabulary, such as "everyday," to express him or herself. This scenario, if frequently repeated, could result in fossilization. In order to overcome fossilization, the learner must notice salient stimuli, and notice his or her own incorrect language production. Furthermore, this noticing must coordinate with motor planning in order to change language behavior.

Noticing; Fossilization and the Five Elements of Attention

In the scenario previously described, influences from procedural memory are greater than those from declarative memory, resulting in the production of a fossilized phrase "Jane walk to school everyday." I propose that the attention process, as outlined in this chapter, accounts for the phenomenon of noticing, as described by Schmidt (1995). Furthermore, I suggest that the many aspects, or elements, of attention can coordinate to correct fossilization in an adult L2 learner (for another discussion of defossilization see chap. 3). To "de-fossilize," (i.e., break the habit of using an over-learned linguistic behavior) I speculate that all of the elements of attention need to be in alignment. Based on all of the previous discussion, these five elements are:

1. **The overall behavioral goal:** For example, a goal to improve L2 speaking.

2. **The task-related goal,** also referred to as the attentional template, or working memory: For example, a goal to change an utterance or execute an utterance with correct grammar.

3. **Motor planning:** For example, planning to adjust or change motor schemata in order to better process environmental stimuli that evoke the grammatically correct response and/or to change and overcome proceduralized motor response plans.

4. **Stimulus qualities:** For example, particularly salient qualities of a stimulus such as, a change in volume, or an unexpected pause in conversation. These stimuli qualities could evoke substantial neural response that would result in a bias strong enough to override a proceduralized response. An internal stimulus, such as a declarative memory, could produce these results as well.

5. **The anterior cingulate:** Assesses the competing influences of the four previous elements.

For defossilization to occur some elements of the attention process have to override predetermined biases from internal stimuli in the form of procedural memory and the motor plans that affect stimuli selection and processing. For example, in order to change, or defossilize, the phrase "Jane walk to school right now," the procedural memory (governed by the basal ganglia) that created the error would have to be influenced by an internal stimulus. This stimulus would be a declarative memory regarding the rule "third person singular takes -s" (see chap. 4, this volume). However, this influence from internal stimuli alone would not be enough to overcome fossilization. Additionally, the motor plans that are activated when the production of third person singular is anticipated would have to have greater influence than the fossilized motor plans.

The interaction of the five elements above may account for noticing as well. Noticing, the awareness of one's speech and language environment, appears necessary to improve learning (Schmidt, 1995). However, noticing does not guarantee learning (Schmidt, 1995). Every learner has experienced situations where he or she is aware of saying an incorrect form but cannot or does not stop the production of that form. For instance, in the example of the learner misusing the simple present, he or she may know (i.e., have stored in declarative memory) that the third person singular requires an "s" but may not be able to coordinate that knowledge with the production of the utterance. I speculate that, in this case, the declarative memory of the correct rule does not create a strong enough bias to override influences from motor plans, procedural memory, and external stimuli. In this scenario, the anterior cingulate weighs the influences of possible responses and actions, and through inhibitory mechanisms, suppresses those with a weaker bias, in this case the influence of a declarative memory. This information is then conveyed via a feedback network to the cortices involved in the continued production of the fossilized phrase. In this manner, a fossilized form which evokes a greater intrinsic neural response could be produced even with the awareness of error. In the example given above, this process could account for the student's ability to be aware of the rule—"third person singular takes morpheme –s." He or she might notice the error in " Jane walk to school every day" during production, but still not be able to correctly execute the phrase. Therefore, noticing, does not ensure changed behavior.

I hypothesize that, during the processing of stimulus/response, the five elements of attention (the overall goal, the task-goal, motor planning, stimulus qualities, and the anterior cingulate) would have to be in continuous alignment in order to fully overcome any existing proceduralized response. However, the five elements are in constant interaction, modulating and refining the processing of stimuli. Thus it is unlikely that alignment would occur frequently. In Fig. 6.7 behavioral and task goals, the DLPFC, motor planning, frontoparietal networks, stimulus qualities, and the anterior cingulate cortex influence each other and bias processing at every step in the refinement of the visual stimulus (i.e., from primary visual cortex, V1, through the most detailed levels of visual processing, V4).

During this refinement, the anterior cingulate is constantly weighing and comparing these influences of the attention elements. Thus, to de-fossilize linguistic behavior, the alignment of all of the five elements of attention would have to be constant throughout stimulus refinement. In an ever-changing environment, this is not likely to occur. This model of de-fossilization could explain why one learner might be receptive to error correction and another might not be (Ellis, 1995; Skehan, 1998). A learner who is receptive to error correction would have sufficient alignment of the elements needed to attend to correction at that time. In order to change fossilized SLA behavior, behavioral goals, task goals, motor planning, and stimulus qualities would have to be in balance, such that the anterior cingulate is presented with compatible response plans—each of which would result in defossilized linguistic behavior.

When the five elements of attention are aligned, a learner notices and changes fossilized habits of language production. Additionally, I speculate that the alignment of these elements produces the noticing often necessary for initial learning, as well as more advanced learning. Some language learners are better at noticing than others (Schmidt, 1995). This difference could

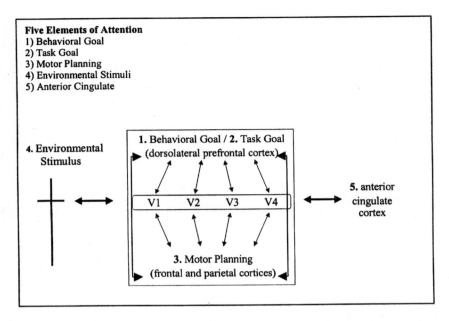

FIG. 6.7. Processing of a visual stimulus and the five elements of attention. This figure illustrates the five elements of attention and the interactive process that creates attentive behavior. In order to change learned behavior, the elements and their influences must be aligned so that no one aspect of the process creates more bias than another. Given the rate of change in the external environment and within the human brain, the alignment of the five elements of attention is uncommon.

be due to several factors, one of which might be a more constant alignment of the attention elements. I suggest three reasons why these learners are more likely to experience alignment. One reason could be that due to personal language learning experience, pathways in the brain have been shaped in a way that allows greater influence of declarative memory on procedural memory (see chap. 3 for a detailed discussion of these pathways). A second reason for increased alignment could be that in the brains of exceptional noticer-learners, the elements of attention are predisposed to alignment. And a third explanation is that both experience influenced pathways and a predisposition for alignment exist in exceptional noticer-learners.

As previously discussed, an additional factor that affects the attention process is motivation. In the appraisal system, Brodmann's area 32 (described as the anterior cingulate by Milham et al., 2001) receives projections influenced by ventral tegmentum (VTA) dopamine via ventromedial ventral pallidum and the mediodorsal thalamus (see chap. 2). In Schumann's discussion of motivation, the anterior cingulate is part of a mechanism for generating mental and motor activity for learning. The present chapter demonstrates that the anterior cingulate weighs biases and influences from goals, stimuli, and motor plans, and sends feedback to cortical areas that shape attentive behavior. Thus, if one combines these functions of the anterior cingulate, it appears that motivation affects the attention process and is possibly woven into the network for optimal performance, the network for attention. As incorporated into the attention process, the anterior cingulate would be affected by structures (amygdala, orbitofrontal cortex, nucleus accumbens) and neuromodulators (e.g., dopamine) involved in appraisal and homeostasis, and then act as the weigh station for influences or biases that generate activity for learning.

CONCLUSION

Attention is just one of many tools necessary for learning. By describing the many neurobiological functions involved in attention it becomes obvious that it is an ongoing, interactive process that defies singular definition. The complexity of attention has been demonstrated in a hypothetical scenario of adult language learning in which the temporal context of the learner and five attentional elements come together to create attentive behavior in a variety of learning situations. Given the interactive qualities and fluid nature of the attention process described here, I reemphasize that the teaching and research literature that refers to attention as a unitary concept, refers to a cultural, psychological concept that is not in the brain. Instead, I have shown that attention is a process involving neurobiology and environment. Some neurobiology is predetermined, such as size and quality of neuronal receptive fields. However, much of neurobiological function is affected by the changing external environment and personal history (i.e. behavioral goals and internal stimuli and memory). The various cortices, functions, and the feedback network that create attentive behavior are part of a complex negotiation between organism and environment.

7   Conclusion

John H. Schumann

In the first chapter, Schumann attempts to give a neurobiological explanation for variation in human mental and physical abilities and for variation in aptitude for second language learning. He argues that all brains are substantially different at the level of microanatomy and physiology. These differences are selected on by the environment and produce vast differences in aptitudes and abilities across human individuals. The goal of this book, as a whole, is to argue that no special mechanisms are required for second language learning, but nevertheless some learners have brains that are so constructed as to give them special talent for acquiring a second language even well after the beneficial effects of a critical or sensitive period would have ceased. This variation in aptitude and the variation in motivation described in the second chapter provide a neurobiological theory for individual differences in second language acquisition and learning in general.

The second chapter proposes a neurobiology for motivation. Arguing that stimulus appraisal underlies motivation (Schumann, 1997), this chapter defined the neurobiological mechanism for such appraisal. Additionally, it proposes neural mechanisms for generating incentive motive or goals, for generating mental and motor activity for learning, for remembering situations or actions to facilitate or predict learning and for laying down memories for language items encountered during learning. This final mechanism—for memory—is elaborated in chapters 3, 4, and 5. Evidence that this neural system actually underlies motivation comes from the literature on drugs of abuse, which co-opt the brain's reward system which was designed by evolution to motivate organisms to take the appropriate motor and mental action to feed and to mate. When humans became a symbolic species, they were able to generate symbolic goals such as the desire to learn a second language. Such symbolic goals operate on the same motivational system that evolved for the basic homeostatic goals of feeding and mating. This picture greatly simplifies the motivation story in second language acquisition. No longer is it necessary to argue about what type of motivation is best for second language learning. What becomes clear is that positive appraisals of stimulus situations in the learning context will generate successful learning to whatever extent the learner's aptitude allows.

Language acquisition, first or second, is profoundly a procedural skill. The third chapter proposes a neurobiology to subserve that skill in second language acquisition. This involved an examination of a neural area that is not typically associated with language and language learning—the basal ganglia. But language use is essentially a motor skill, and therefore, we hypothesized that the basal ganglia, as a major component of the nonpyramidal motor system, is involved in adult second language acquisition. Lee (chap. 3) suggested that the direct pathways in the basal ganglia subserve the execution of L2 structures whereas the indirect pathways subserve inhibition of L1 structures. Fossilization is a major issue in second language learning, and based on Wu (2000), Lee's model argued that fossilization involves the premature proceduralization of incompletely learned L2 forms. But repetition of incorrect forms does not always lead to fossilization, and Lee argued that this result may have to do with dopamine strengthening of the circuits for correct forms and the intervention of declarative knowledge. Additionally, fossilized forms sometimes can defossilize. To account for these phenomena, this chapter suggests a neural mechanism that allows declarative knowledge to influence and become procedural knowledge and also proposes that this same system allows declarative knowledge of correct rules to influence and remediate fossilized structures encoded in the basal ganglia system for procedural knowledge.

In the fourth chapter, Crowell lays out the anatomical and cellular bases for memory formation. Within that framework, she offers several important hypotheses about how the hippocampal formation in general and long-term potentiation in particular may be involved in second language learning. She provides a model for how explicitly taught grammar rules and lexical items are cycled through the various components of the hippocampal structure to establish LTP for these items and thus to initiate them in memory. With respect to declarative versus procedural learning, Crowell hypothesized that what is seen as a conversion of declarative knowledge to procedural skill may in fact be a strengthening of connections in the basal ganglia circuitry through practice (guided by declarative knowledge) and a concomitant weakening in the hippocampal circuits as the basal ganglia takes over. Crowell also made the interesting speculation that individual variation in gene processes that produce CREB and C/EBP that convert short-term memories into long-term memories may underlie the variations seen among second language learners in the ability to acquire target language lexical items rapidly.

Jones, in the fifth chapter, explores the neurobiology underlying the long-term goal of second language acquisition, that is, the consolidation of memories such that L2 knowledge will be available on a permanent basis. In this effort, she follows the tenets of Multiple Trace Theory, which she relates to Pulvermüller's Cortical Cell Assembly Theory to suggest a model of second language acquisition in which there are no special mechanisms or locations in the brain that specially subserve the L2 lexicon. She also proposes how Multiple Trace Theory might effect individual differences in learning and how that theory is relevant to research done on bilinguals and aphasics. Finally, her account stresses the importance of context in all hippocampal learning and applies that account to second language acquisition.

Schuchert wrestles with an extremely important and very frequently unrecognized problem. The issue is whether mechanisms proposed in psychology by working backward from behavior are appropriate when attempting to define brain mechanisms. *Attention* is just such a term. It has been inferred by psychologists as a mechanism to explain certain behavioral phenomena, but one has to ask whether the term can be directly mapped onto the brain. Schuchert examines this issue by exploring the relationship of the concept of attention to a multitude of processes that have been ascribed to the brain. She explores whether attention at the level of the brain is different from intention, from perception, from action response, from goals, or from working memory. She then hypothesizes five neural components of attention and to shows how they apply to the problems of defossilization and "noticing" in second language acquisition.

The following Fig. 7.1 brings together all the neural areas that we have discussed in relation to second language acquisition. In fact, the anatomy depicted in the figure involves nearly all major areas of the brain. There would appear to be no module for second language acquisition. Indeed, there would appear to be no module for even grammar in second language acquisition. Our analysis of the components of SLA (motivation, procedural skill, declarative knowledge, and attention) requires the whole brain. A major orientation in SLA is universal grammar (UG). But it appears there is no neural biological substrate that constitutes a UG for the acquisition of a second language. The neural equipment for every aspect of the SLA process is available in general learning systems distributed throughout the brain. From this perspective, the acquisition of the second language by an adult learner is like the acquisition of any other knowledge or skill. What it would mean to have partial access to UG in

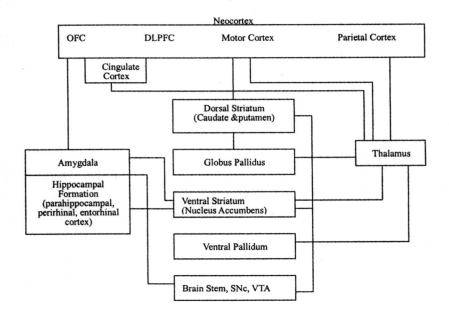

Motivation	Procedural Knowledge	Declarative Knowledge and Memory consolidation	Attention
OFC, Amygdala, Ventral Striatum, SNc, VTA	Dorsal Striatum, Globus Pallidus, Thalamus, Motor ctx	Hippocampal Formation, Neocortex	DLPFC, Parietal ctx, Anterior Cingulate (Inter Alia)

FIG. 7.1. The neural substrate for SLA.

second language acquisition is totally opaque from the neurobiological perspective. The UG claim is a neurobiological claim; it is a theory of the brain, but as is argued in this book, the neural mechanisms to subserve the acquisition of a second language exist to subserve learning in general. Of course, there maybe an emergent UG from the interactions of these various components, but we do not see it yet.

If our thinking about second language learning is not constrained by the biology of learning, and if it is only constrained by an analysis of the product of that learning, then we can say almost anything about underlying mechanisms. As mentioned in the introduction, we can invoke, as though they were real, mechanisms such as an affective filter, cognitive operating principles, noticing, monitoring, pidginization, nativization, cognitive strategies, and learning strategies. But in the 21st century, after years of brain research that actually allows us to consider neural processes in language acquisition should we limit ourselves to metaphors? It is our view that we should not. We can constrain our metaphors with biological knowledge. But only a handful of people in our field have that knowledge. However, this need not be the case. Neurobiology is learnable and serious programs in second language acquisition will find ways for their students to learn it. A recent issue of *The Annual Review of Applied Linguistics* (2001) dealt with the relationship between applied linguistics and psychology. This issue was published some 25 years after the founding of the American Association for Applied Linguistics. Second language acquisition is a subfield of Applied Linguistics and is as much psychological as it is linguistic. But just as we are making our links with psychology, psychology is becoming radically biologized. Psychological biology is something all students of psychology study these days. Will it be 2030 before the *Annual Review of Applied Linguistics* initiates a connection with neurobiology? Can we always afford to be 25 years behind the times?

Neural imaging technology such as PET and fMRI are generating pictures of the brain which are appearing daily in popular magazines, newspapers and on television programs. This technology, which is essential for the medical profession, is going to continue to drive research in neurobiology. Researchers have already begun stuffing human second language learners into those machines, and pictures of brain activation during second language use are appearing. What are we to make of these pictures? How are we to interpret them? One of the worst things that could happen is that the field as a whole learns its neurobiology by what shows up those pictures. It should happen the other way around. Second language acquisition researchers should know enough neurobiology to form hypotheses about what would be activated during various kinds of second language behavior, and then they should test these hypotheses with imaging research. The basal ganglia, which features so importantly in our discussion of second language acquisition, is rarely considered a language area. Therefore, without some a priori notion that the basal ganglia should subserve procedural skill in SLA, we would either not look for, not find, or would ignore basal ganglia activation in research related to language learning. Our field had better be prepared to evaluate neural imaging research involving second language acquisition or it will be forced to turn over authority for interpretations to those who do not understand SLA.

References

Adolphs, R., & Tranel, D. (1999). Preferences for visual stimuli following amygdala damage. *Journal of Cognitive Neuroscience, 11,* 610–616.

Adolphs, R., Tranel, D., & Damasio, A. R. (1998). The human amygdala in social judgment. *Nature, 393,* 470–474.

Adolphs, R., Tranel, D., Damasio, H., & Damasio, A. R. (1994). Impaired recognition of emotion in facial expressions following bilateral damgage to the human amygdala. *Nature, 372,* 669–672.

Aglioti, S. (1999). Language and memory systems. In F. Fabbro (Ed.), *Concise encyclopedia of language pathology* (pp. 371–377). Oxford: Pergaman Press.

Aglioti, S., Beltramello, A., Girardi, F., & Fabbro, F. (1996). Neurolinguistic and follow-up study of an unusual pattern of recovery from bilingual subcortical aphasia. *Brain, 119,* 1551–1564.

Aglioti, S., & Fabbro, F. (1993). Paradoxical selective recovery in a bilingual aphasic following subcortical lesions. *Neuroreport, 4,* 1359–1362.

Anderson, S. W., Bechara, A., Damasio, H., Tranel, D., & Damasio, A. R. (1999). Impairment of social and moral behavior related to early damage in human prefrontal cortex. *Nature Neuroscience, 2,* 1032–1037.

Awh, E., & Jonides, J. (1998). Spatial working memory and spatial selective attention. In R. Parasuraman (Ed.), *The attentive brain* (pp. 95–122). Cambridge, MA: MIT Press.

Bailey, C. H., Bartsch, D., & Kandel, E. R. (1996). Toward a molecular definition of long-term memory storage. *Proceedings of the National Academy of Sciences, USA, 93,* 13445–13452.

Bailey, C. H., & Kandel, E. R. (1993). Structural changes accompanying memory storage. *Annual Review of Physiology, 55,* 397–426.

Baranyi, A., Szente, M. B., & Woody, C. D. (1991). Properties of associative long-lasting potentiation induced by cellular conditioning in the motor cortex of conscious cats. *Neuroscience, 42*(2), 321–334.

Bardo, M. T. (1998). Neuropharmacological mechanisms of drug reward: Beyond dopamine in the nucleus accumbens. *Critical Reviews in Neurobiology, 12*(1&2), 37–67.

Bartley, A. J., Jones, D. W., & Weinberger, D. R. (1997). Genetic variability of human brain size cortical gyral patterns. *Brain, 120,* 257–269.

Baxter, M. G., & Murray, A. M. (2002). The amygdala and reward. *Nature Reviews Neuroscience, 3,* 563–573.

Bechara, A., Damasio, H., & Damasio, A. R. (2000). Emotion, decision making and the orbitofrontal cortex. *Cerebral Cortex, 10,* 295–307.

Benes, F. M. (1993). Relationship of cortex to schizophrenia and other psychiatric disorders. In B. A. Vogt, & M. Gabriel (Eds.), *Neurobiology of cingulate cortex and limbic thalamus* (pp. 581–605). New York: Birkhauser.

Berry, D. C. (1994). Implicit and explicit learning of complex tasks. In N. C. Ellis (Ed.), *Implicit and explicit learning of languages* (pp. 147–164). San Diego, CA: Academic Press.

Bliss, T. V., & Lømo, T. (1973). Long-lasting potentiation of synaptic transmission in the dentate area of the anaesthetized rabbit following stimulation of the perforant path. *Journal of Physiology, 232,* 331–356.

Bliss, T. V. P., & Collingridge, G. L. (1993). A synaptic model of memory: Long-term potentiation in the hippocampus. *Nature, 361,* 31–39.

Blumstein, S. E., Alexander, M. P., Ryalls, J. H., Katz, W., & Dworetzky, B. (1987). On the nature of the foreign accent syndrome: A case study. *Brain and Language, 31,* 215–244.

Bonda, E., Petrides, M., Ostry, O., & Evans, A. (1996). Specific involvement of human parietal systems and the amygdala in the perception of biological motion. *Journal of Neuroscience, 16,* 3737–3744.

Botvinick, M. M., Nystrom, L. E., Fissell, K., Carter, C. S., & Cohen, J. D. (1999). Conflict monitoring versus selection-for-action in anterior cingulate cortex. *Nature, 402,* 179–180.

Braun, J. (1998). Divided attention: Narrowing the gap between brain and behavior. In R. Parasuraman (Ed.), *The attentive brain* (pp. 95–122). Cambridge, MA: MIT Press.

Brothers, L. (1995). Neurophysiology of the perception of intentions by primates. In M. S. Gazzaniga (Ed.), *The cognitive neurosciences* (pp. 1107–1115). Cambridge, MA: MIT Press.

Brown, E. N., Frank, L. M., Tang, D., Quirk, M. C., & Wilson, M. A. (1998). A statistical paradigm for neural spike train decoding applied to position prediction from ensemble firing patterns of rat hippocampal place cells. *Journal of Neuroscience, 18,* 7411–7425

Brown, T. H., Chapman, P. F., Kairiss, E. W., & Keenan, C. L. (1988). Long-term synaptic potentiation. *Science, 242*(4879), 724–729.

Calvin, W. H. (1996). *How brains think.* New York: Basic Books.

Cameron, K. A., Yashar, S., Wilson, C. L., & Fried, I. (2001). Human hippocampal neurons predict how well word pairs will be remembered. *Neuron, 30,* 289–298.

Caramazza, A., & Shelton, J. R. (1998). Domain-specific knowledge systems in the brain: the animate-inanimate distinction. *Journal of Cognitive Neuroscience, 10,* 1–34.

Carlson, N. R. (2001). *Physiology of behavior.* Boston, MA: Pearson Education.

Carroll, J. B., & Sapon, S. (1959). *Modern language aptitude test—Form A.* New York. The Psychological Corporation.

Carter, C. S., Braver, T. S., Barch, D. M., Botvinick, M. M., Noll, D., & Cohen, J. D. (1998). Anterior cingulate cortex, error detection, and the online monitoring of performance. *Science, 280,* 747–749.

Celce-Murcia, M., Brinton, D. M., & Goodwin, J. M. (1996). *Teaching pronunciation: A reference for teachers of English to speakers of other languages.* Cambridge, UK: Cambridge University Press.

Chao, L., Haxby, J. V., & Martin, A. (1999). Attribute-based neural substrates in temporal cortex for perceiving and knowing about objects. *Nature Neuroscience, 2,* 913–919.

Chao L., & Martin, A. (1999). Cortical representation of perception, naming, and knowing about color. *Journal of Cognitive Neuroscience, 11,* 25–35.

Chen, H. (1990). Lexical processing in a non-native language: Effects of language proficiency and learning strategy. *Memory and Cognition, 18*(3), 279–288.

Cho, Y. H., Beracochea, D., & Jaffard, R. (1993). Extended temporal gradient for the retrograde and anterograde amnesia produced by ibotenate entorhinal cortex lesions in mice. *Journal of Neuroscience, 13*(4), 1759–1766.

Chrobak, J. J., Lorincz, A., & Buzsaki, G. (2000). Physiological patterns in the hippocampo-entorhinal cortex system. *Hippocampus, 10*(4), 457–465.

Clarke, P. B. S. (1991). The mesolimbic dopamine system as a target for nicotine. In F. Adlkofer & K. Thurau (Eds.), *Effects of nicotine on biological systems*. Berlin: Birkhauser Verlag.

Clement, R., Dornyei, Z., & Noels, K. A. (1994). Motivation, self-confidence, and group cohesion in the foreign language classroom. *Language Learning, 44,* 417–448.

Constantinidis, C., Williams, G. V., & Goldman-Rakic, P. S. (2002). A role for inhibition in shaping the temporal flow of information in prefrontal cortex. *Nature Neuroscience, 5*(2) 175–180.

Corbetta, M. (1998). Functional anatomy of visual attention in the human brain: Studies with positron emission tomography. In R. Parasuraman (Ed.), *The attentive brain* (pp. 95–122). Cambridge, MA: MIT Press.

Corbetta, M., & Schulman, G. L. (2002). Control of goal-directed and stimulus-driven attention in the brain. *Nature Reviews Neuroscience, 3,* 201–215.

Corrigal, W. A. (1991). Regulation of intravenous nicotine self-administration—dopamine mechanisms. In F. Adlkofer & K. Thurau (Eds.), *Effects of nicotine on biological systems* (pp. 423–432). Berlin: Birkhauser Verlag.

Csikszentmihalyi, M., & Larson, R. (1987). Validity and reliability of the experience-sampling method. *The Journal of Nervous and Mental Disease, 175,* 526–536.

Csikszentmihalyi, M., Rathunde, K., & Wholen, S. (1993). *Talented teens: The roots of success and failure*. New York: Cambridge University Press.

Damasio, A. R., & Damasio, H. (1992). Brain and language. *Scientific American, 267*(3), 88–95.

Damasio, A. R. (1994). *Descartes' error: Emotion, reason, and the human brain*. New York: G.P. Putnam's Sons.

Damasio, H., Grabowski, T., Tranel, D., & Hichwa, R. (1996). A neural basis for lexical retrieval. *Nature, 380*(6574), 499–505.

Deacon, T. W. (1997). *The symbolic species: The co-evolution of language and the brain*. New York: W. W. Norton & Company.

DeKeyser, R. M. (1997). Beyond explicit rule learning. *Studies in Second Language Acquisition, 19,* 195–221.

Desimone, R. & Duncan, J. (1995). Neural mechanisms of selective visual attention. *Annual Reviews Neuroscience, 18,* 193–222.

Deutch, A. Y., Bourdelais, A. J., & Zahm, D. S. (1993). The nucleus accumbens core and shell: Accumbal compartments and their functional attributes. In P. W. Kalivas & C. D. Barnes (Eds.), *Limbic motor circuits and neuropsychiatry* (pp. 45–88). Boca Raton, FL: CRC Press.

Diamond, M. C., Scheibel, A. B., Murphy, J. G. M., & Harvey, T. (1985). On the brain of a scientist: Albert Einstein. *Experimental Neurology, 88,* 198–204.

DiChiara, G. (1995). The role of dopamine in drug abuse viewed from the perspective of its role in motivation. *Drug and Alcohol Dependence, 38,* 95–137.

DiChiara, G., Acquas, E., Tanda, G., & Cadoni, C. (1993). Drugs of abuse: Biochemical surrogates of specific aspects of natural reward? *Biochemical Society Symposium, 59,* 65–81.

DiChiara, G., & Imperato, A. (1988). Drugs abused by humans preferentially increase synaptic dopamine concentrations in the mesolimbic system of freely moving rats. *Proceedings of the National Academy of Science of the United States of America 85,* 5274.

Dolan, R. J., & Fletcher, P. F. (1999). Encoding and retrieval in human medial temporal lobes: An empirical investigation using functional magnetic resonance imaging (fMRI). *Hippocampus, 9,* 25–34.

Driver, J., & Baylis, G. C. (1998). Attention and visual object segmentation. In R. Parasuraman (Ed.), *The attentive brain* (pp. 95–122). Cambridge, MA: MIT Press.

Driver, J., & Frith, C. D. (2000). Shifting baselines in attention research. *Nature Reviews Neuroscience, 1,* 147–148.

Duncan, J., & Owen, A. M. (2000). Common regions of the human frontal lobe recruited by diverse cognitive demands. *Trends in Neuroscience, 23,* 475–483.

Dunn, J., & Plomin, R. (1990). *Separate lives: Why siblings are so different.* New York: Basic Books.

DuPont, R. L. (1997). *The selfish brain: Learning from addiction.* Washington, DC: American Psychiatric Press.

Edelman, G. M. (1987). *Neural Darwinism: The theory of neuronal group selection.* New York: Basic Books.

Edelman, G. M. (1989). *The remembered present.* New York: Basic Books.

Edelman, G. M. (1992). *Bright air brilliant fire: On the matter of mind.* New York: Basic Books.

Edelman, G. M., & Tononi, G. (2000). *A universe of consciousness.* New York: Basic Books.

Eichenbaum, H., & Bodkin, J. A. (1999). Belief and knowledge as distinct forms of memory. In D. Schacter & E. Scarry (Eds.), *Memory, brain and belief* (pp. 176–207). Cambridge, MA: Harvard University Press.

Ellis, R. (1994). *The study of second language acquisition.* Oxford: Oxford University press.

Ellis, R. (2000). *Second language acquisition* (Oxford introductions to language study). Oxford: Oxford University Press.

Eubank, L., & Gregg, K. R. (1995). "Et in amygdala ego": UG, (S)LA and neurobiology. *Studies in Second Language Acquisition, 17,* 35–57.

Fabbro, F. (1999). *The neurolinguistics of bilingualism: An introduction.* Hove, UK: Psychology Press.

Fabbro, F., & Asher, R. E. (1999). *Concise encyclopedia of language pathology.* Oxford: Pergamon Press.

Fabbro, F., & Paradis, M. (1995a). Acquired aphasia in a bilingual child. In M. Paradis (Ed.), *Aspects of bilingual aphasia* (pp. 67–83). London: Pergamon Press.

Fabbro, F., & Paradis, M. (1995b). Differential impairments in four multilingual patients with subcortical lesions. In M. Paradis (Ed), *Aspects of bilingual aphasia* (pp. 139–176). London: Pergamon Press.

Fadiga, L., Fogassi, L., Gallese, V., & Rizzolatti, G. (2000). Visuomotor neurons: Ambiguity of the discharge or "motor" perception? *International Journal of Psychophysiology, 35*(2–3), 165–177.

Fanselow, M., & LeDoux, J. (1999). Why we think plasticity underlying Pavlovian fear conditioning occurs in the basolateral amygdala. *Neuron, 23*(2), 229–32.

Fernández, G., Brewer, J. B., Zhao, Z., Glover, G. H., & Gabrieli, J. D. E. (1999). Level of sustained entorhinal activity at study correlates with subsequent cued-recall performance: A functional magnetic resonance imaging study with high acquisition rate. *Hippocampus, 9,* 35–44.

Fernández, G., Weyerts, H., Schrader-Bolsche, M., Tendolkar, I., Smid, H. G. O. M., Tempelmann, C., Hinrichs, H., Scheich, H., Elger, C. E., Mangun, G. R., & Heinze, H.-J. (1998). Successful verbal encoding into episodic memory engages the posterior hippocampus: A parametrically analyzed functional magnetic resonance imaging study. *Journal of Neuroscience, 18*(5), 1841–1847.

Ferry, B., Roozendaal, B., & McGaugh, J. (1999). Role of norepinephrine in mediating stress hormone regulation of long-term memory storage: A critical involvement of the amygdala. *Society of Biological Psychiatry, 46,* 1140–1152.

de Fockert, J.W., Rees, G., Frith, C. D., & Lavie, N. (2001). The role of working memory in visual selective attention. *Science, 291,* 1803–1806.

Frijda, N. H. (1987). Emotion, cognitive structures and action tendency. *Cognition & Emotion, 1,* 115–144.

Frijda, N. H., Knipers, P., & ter Schure, E. (1989). Relations among emotion, appraisal, and emotional action readiness. *Journal of Personality and Social Psychology, 57,* 212–228.

Friston, K. J., Tononi, G., Reek Jr., G. N., Sporns, O., & Edelman, G. M. (1994). Value-dependent selection in the brain: Simulation in a sythetic neural model. *Neuroscience, 59,* 229–243.

Funehashi, S., Bruce, C.J., & Goldman-Rakic, P. S. (1990). Visuospatial coding in primate prefrontal neurons revealed by oculomotor paradigms. *Journal of Neurophysiology, 63,* 814–831.

Fuster, J. M. (1995). *Memory in the cerebral cortex.* Cambridge, MA: MIT Press.

Fuster, J. M. (1996). Frontal lobe and the cognitive foundation of behavioral action. In A. R. Damasio, H. Damasio, & Y. Christen (Eds.), *Neurobiology of decision-making* (pp. 47–61) Berlin Heidelberg: Springer-Verlag.

Fuster, J. (1999). Hebb's other postulate at work on words. *Behavior and Brain Sciences, 22,* 288–289.

Gallistel, C. R. (1995). Is long-term potentiation a plausible basis for memory? In J. L. McGaugh, N. M. Weinberger, & G. Lynch (Eds.), *Brain and memory* (pp. 328–337). New York: Oxford University Press.

Gardner, H. (1993). *Frames of mind.* New York: Basic Books.

Gardner, H. (1999). *Intelligence reframed.* New York: Basic Books.

Gardner, R. (1985). *Social psychology and second language learning: The role of attitudes and motivation.* London: Edward Arnold.

Gehm, T., & Scherer, K. R. (1988). Relating situation evaluation to emotion differentiation: Nonmetric analysis of cross-cultural questionnaire data. In K. R. Scherer (Ed.), *Facets of emotion: Recent research* (pp. 61–77). Hillsdale, NJ: Lawrence Erlbaum Associates.

Geinisman, Y. (2000). Structural synaptic modifications associated with hippocampal LTP and behavioral learning. *Cerebral Cortex, 10*(10), 952–962.

Genesee, F. (1988). Neuropsychology and second language acquisition. *Issues in Second Language Acquisition.* Boston, MA: Heinle & Heinle.

Gessa, G. C., Muntoni, F., Cullu, M., Vargiu, L., & Mereu, G. (1985). Low doses of ethanol activate dopaminergic neurons in the ventral tegmental area. *Brain Research, 348,* 201–203.

Gilmore, R. O., & Johnson, M. H. (1995). Working memory in six-month-old infants revealed by versions of the oculomotor delayed response task. *Journal of Experimental Child Psychology, 59,* 397–418.

Gluck, M., & Meyers, C. (1998). Hippocampal Function in Learning and Memory. *Neurobiology of learning and memory* (pp. 417–488). San Diego: Academic Press.

Graybiel, A. M. (1998). The basal ganglia and chunking of action repertoires. *Neurobiology of learning and memory, 70,* 119–136.

Graybiel, A. M., Aosaki, T., Flaherty, A. W., & Kimura, M. (1994). The basal ganglia and adaptive motor control. *Science, 265,* 1826–1831.

Gurd, J. M., Bessell, N. J., Bladon, R. A. W., & Bamford, J. M. (1988). A case of foreign accent syndrom, with follow-up clinical, neuropsychological and phonetic descriptions. *Neuropsychologia, 26*(2), 237–251.

Haiman, J. (1983). Iconic and economic motivation. *Language, 59*(4).

Halpern, L. (1941). Restitution in polyglot aphasia with regard to Hebrew. Translated in M. Paradis (Ed.), (1983). *Readings on aphasia in bilinguals and polyglots* (pp. 418–422). Montreal: Didier.

Hamann, S. B., Ely, T. D., Grafton, S. T., & Kilts, C. D. (1999). Amygdala activity related to enhanced memory for pleasant and aversive stimuli. *Nature Neuroscience, 2,* 289–293.

Hamer, D., & Copeland, P. (1998). *Living with our genes.* New York: Anchor Books.

Harley, B., & Swain, M. (1978). An analysis of the verb system by young learners of French. *Interlanguage Studies Bulletin, 3*(1), 35–79.

Hebb, D. O. (1949). *The organization of behavior; a neuropsychological theory.* Oxford, England: Wiley.

Heimer, L., Alheid, G. F., & Zahm, D. S. (1993). The basal forebrain organization: An anatomical framework for motor aspects of drive and motivation. In P. W. Kalivas & C. D. Barnes (Eds.), *Limbic motor circuits and neuorpsychiatry* (pp. 1–43). Boca Raton, FL: CRC Press.

Heun, R., Jessen, F., Klose, U., Erb, M., Granath, D. O., & Grodd, W. (2000). Response-related fMRI analysis during encoding and retrieval revealed differences in cerebral activation by retrieval success. *Psychiatry Research: Neuroimaging Section, 99,* 137–150.

Hikosaka, O., Miyashita, K., Miyachi, S., Sakai, K., & Lu, X. (1998). Differential roles of the frontal cortex, basal ganglia, and the cerebellum in visuomotor sequence learning. *Neurobiology of Learning and Memory, 70,* 137–149.

Hikosaka, O., Nakahara, H., Rand, M. K., Sakai, K., Lu, X., Nakamura, K., Miyachi, S., & Doya, K. (1999). Parallel neural networks for learning sequential procedurea. *Trends in Neuroscience, 22,* 464–471.

Hikosaka, O., Rand, M. K., Miyachi, S., & Miyashita, K. (1995). Learning of sequential movements in the monkey: Process of learning and retention of memory. *Journal of Neurophysiology, 74,* 1652–1661.

Hikosaka, O., Sakai, K., Miyauchi, S., Takino, R., Sasaki, Y., & Putz, B. (1996). Activation of human presupplementary motor area in learning of sequential procedures: A functional MRI study. *Journal of Neurophysiology, 76,* 617–621.

Hoshi, E., & Tanji, J. (2000). Integration of target and body-part information in the premotor cortex when planning action. *Nature, 408,* 466–470.

Houk, J. C., Adams, J. L., & Barto, A. G. (1995a). A model of how the basal ganglia generate and use neural signals that predict reinforcement. In J. C. Houk, J. L. Davis, & D. G. Beiser (Eds.), *Models of information processing in the basal ganglia* (pp. 249–170). Cambridge, MA : MIT Press.

Houk, J. C., Davis, J. L., & Beiser, D. G. (Eds.). (1995b). *Models of information processing in the basal ganglia.* Cambridge, MA: MIT Press.

Hurd, Y. L. (1996). Cocaine effects on dopamine and opioid peptide neural systems: Implications for humna cocaine abuse. In M. D. Majewska (Ed.), *Neurotoxicity and neuropathology associated with cocaine abuse.* Rockville, MD: National Institutes of Health.

Huston-Lyons, D., & Kornetsky, C. (1992). Brain-stimulation reward as a model of drug-induced euphoria: Comparison of cocaine and opiates. In J. M. Lakoski, M. P. Galloway, & F. J. White (Eds.), *Cocaine: Pharmacology, physiology and clinical strategies.* Boca Raton, FL: CRC Press.

Iacoboni, M. (2000). Attention and sensorimotor integration *mapping the embodied mind.* In A. Toga, & J. Mazziotta, (Eds.) *Brain mapping: The systems.* San Diego, CA: Academic Press.

Ikemoto, S., & Panksepp, J. (1999). The role of nucleus accumbens dopamine in motivated behavior: A unifying interpretation with special reference to reward-seeking. *Brain Research Reviews, 31*(1), 6–41.

Jacobs, B. (1988). Neurobiological differentiation of primary and secondary language acquisition. *Studies in Second Language Acquisition, 10,* 303–337.

Jacobs, B., & Schumann, J. (1992). Language acquisition and the neurosciences: Towards a more integrative perspective. *Applied Linguistics, 13,* 282–301.

James, W. (1950). *The principles of psychology.* Oxford, England: Dover Publications.

Joel, D., & Weiner, I. (1998). Striatal contention scheduling and the split circuit scheme of basal ganglia-thalamocortical circuitry: From anatomy to behavior. In R. Miller, & J. R. Wickens (Eds.) *Conceptual advances in brain research: Brain dynamics and the striatal complex* (pp. 209–236). Amsterdam: Harwood Academic Publishers.

Jog, M. S., Kubota, Y., Connolly, C. I., Hillegaart, V., & Graybiel, A. M. (1999). Building neural representations of habits. *Science, 286,* 1745–1749.

Johnson, M.I. (1998). Developing an attentive brain. In R. Parasuraman (Ed.), *The attentive brain* (pp. 95–122). Cambridge, MA: MIT Press.

Johnson, S. C., Saykin, A. J., Flashman, L. A., McAllister, T. W., & Sparling, M. B. (2001). Brain activation on fMRI and verbal memory ability: Functional neuroanatomic correlates of CVLT performance. *Journal of the International Neuropsychological Society, 7*, 55–62.

Jueptner, M., Frith, C. D., Brooks, D. J., Frackowiak, R. S. J., & Passingham, R. E. (1997). Anatomy of motor learning II: Subcortical structures and learning by trial and error. *Journal of Neurophysiology, 77*, 1325–1337.

Jueptner, M., Stephan, K. M., Frith, C. D., Brooks, D. J., Frackowiak, R. S. J., & Passingham, R. E. (1997). Anatomy of motor learning. I: Frontal cortex and attention to action. *Journal of Neurophysiology, 77*, 1313–1324.

Kaas, J. H., & Hackett, T. A. (1999). "What" and "where" processing in auditory cortex. *Nature Neuroscience, 2*(12), 1045–1047.

Kalivas, P. W., Churchill, L., & Klitenick, M. A. (1993). The circuitry mediating the translation of motivational stimuli into adaptive motor responses. In P. W. Kalivas & C. D. Barnes (Eds.), *Limbic motor circuits and neuropsychiatry* (pp. 237–287). Boca Raton, FL: CRC Press.

Kandel, E., Schwartz, J., & Jessell, T. (2000). *Principles of neural science* (4th ed.). New York: McGraw-Hill.

Kanwisher, N., & Wojciulik, E. (2000). Visual attention: insights from brain imaging. *Nature Reviews Neuroscience, 1*, 91–100.

Kawagoe, R., Takikawa, Y., & Hikosaka, O. (1998). Expectation of reward modulates cognitive signals in the basal ganglia. *Nature Neuroscience, 1*(5), 411–416.

Kim, J. J., & Fanselow, M. S. (1992). Modality-specific retrograde amnesia of fear. *Science, 256*(5057), 675–677.

Kim, K., Relkin, N., Lee, K., & Hirsch, J. (1997). Distinct cortical areas associated with native and second languages. *Nature, 388*, 171–174.

Kimura, M., & Graybiel, A. M. (1995). Role of basal ganglia in sensory motor association learning. In M. Kimura, & A. M. Graybiel (Eds.), *Functions of the cortico-basal ganglia loop* (pp. 2–17). New York: Springer-Verlag.

Klein, D., Zatorre, R. J., Milner, B., Evans, A. C., & Meyer, E. (1994). Left putaminal activation when speaking a second language: evidence from PET. *Neuroreport, 5*, 2295–2297.

Klein, D., Zatorre, R. J., Milner, B., Meyer, E., & Evans, A. C. (1995). The neural substrates of bilingual language processing: Evidence from positron emission tomography. In M. Paradis (Ed.), *Aspects of bilingual aphasia* (pp. 23–36). London: Pergamon.

Kohler, S., Moscovitch, M., Wincour, G., & McIntosh, A. (2000). Episodic encoding and recognition of pictures and words: role of the human medial temporal lobes. *Acta Psychologica, 105*, 159–179.

Koob, G. F., & Nestler, E. J. (1997). The neurobiology of addiction. *The Journal of Neuropsychiatry and clinical Neuroscience, 9*, 482–497.

Krashen, S. (1977). Some issues relating to the monitor model. In H. Brown, C. Yorio, & R. Crymes (Eds.), *On TESOL, 77* (pp. 144–158). Washington, DC: Teachers of English to Speakers of Other Languages.

Krashen, S. (1982). *Principles and practice in second language acquisition.* New York: Pergamon Press.

Krashen, S. (1985). *The input hypothesis: Issues and implications.* New York: Longman.

Krashen, S. (1994). The input hypothesis and its rivals. In N. C. Ellis (Ed.), *Implicit and explicit learning of languages* (pp. 45–78). San Diego, CA: Academic Press.

Krashen, S. (1995). *Principles and practice in second language acquisition.* Hertford-shire, UK: Phoenix ELT.

Kreiman, G., Koch, C., & Fried, I. (2000). Category-specific visual responses of single neurons in the human medial temporal lobe. *Nature Neuroscience, 3,* 946–953.

Kroll, J., & de Groot, A. (1997). Lexical and conceptual memory in the bilingual: mapping form to meaning in two languages. In A. de Groot & J. Kroll (Eds.) *Tutorials in bilingualism: Psycholinguistic perspectives* (pp. 169–199). Mahwah, NJ: Lawrence Erlbaum Associates.

Kuno, M. (1995). *The synapse: Function plasticity, and neurotrophism.* New York: Oxford Universtiy Press.

LaBerge, D. (1995). *Attention processing: The brain's art of mindfulness.* Cambridge, MA: Harvard University Press.

Lamendella, J. T. (1977). General principles of neurofunctional organization and their manifestation in primary and nonprimary language acquisition. *Language Learning, 27,* 155–196.

Laroche, S., Davis, S., & Jay, T. M. (2000). Plasticity at hippocampal to prefrontal cortex synapses: Dual roles in working memory and consolidation. *Hippocampus, 10,* 438–446.

Larsen-Freeman, D., & Long, M. (1991). *An introduction to second language acquisition research.* London: Longman.

Lawrence, A. D., Sahakian, B. J., & Robbins, T. (1998). Cognitive functions and corticostriatal circuits: Insights from Huntington's disease. *Trends in Cognitive Sciences, 2*(10), 379–388.

LeDoux, J. (1996). *The emotional brain.* New York: Simon & Schuster.

Lemley, B. (2000). Isn't she lovely. *Discover, 21,* 41–49.

Lenneberg, E. H. (1967). *Biological foundations of language.* Marlabar, FL: Robert E. Krieger Publishing Company.

Lepage, M., Habib, R., & Tulving, E. (2000). Hippocampal PET activations of memory encoding and retrieval: the HIPER model. *Hippocampus, 8,* 313–322.

Leventhal, H. (1984). A perceptual-motor theory of emotion. In L. Berkowitz (Ed.), *Advances in Experimental Social Psychology, 17,* 117–182. New York: Academic Press.

Leventhal, H., & Scherer, K. (1987). The relationship of emotion to cognition: A functional approach to a semantic controversy. *Cognition & Emotion, 1,* 3–28.

Levelt, W. (1989). *Speaking: From intention to articulation.* Cambridge, MA: MIT Press.

Liang, K., Juler, R., & McGaugh, J. (1986). Modulating effects of posttraining epinephrine on memory: Involvement of the amygdala noradrenergic system. *Brain Research, 368*(1). 125–133.

Lieberman, P. (2000). *Human language and our reptilian brain.* Cambridge, MA: Harvard University Press.

Lieberman, P., Kako, E., Friedman, J., Tajchman, G., Feldman, L. S., & Jiminez, E. B. (1992). Speech production, syntax comprehension, and cognitive deficits in Parkinson's disease. *Brain and Language, 43*(2), 169–189.

Littlewood, W. (1994). *Foreign and second language learning.* Cambridge, UK: Cambridge University Press.

Locke, J. L. (1995). Development of the capacity for spoken language. In P. F. Fletcher & B. MacWhinney (Eds.), *The handbook of child language* (pp. 278–302). Oxford, UK: Blackwell.

Loftus, E., Miller, D., & Burns, H. (1978). Semantic integration of verbal information into a visual memory. *Journal of Experimental Psychology: Human Learning and Memory, 4*(1), 19–31.

Loftus, E., & Pickrell, J. (1995). The formation of false memories. *Psychiatric Annals, 25*(12), 720–725.

Long, M. H. (1990). The least a second language acquisition theory needs to explain. *TESOL Quarterly, 24,* 649–666.

Lotto, L., & de Groot, A. (1998). Effects of learning method and word type on acquiring vocabulary in an unfamiliar language. *Language Learning, 48*(1), 31–69.

Louie, K., & Wilson, M. A. (2001). Temporally structured replay of awake hippocampal ensemble activity during rapid eye movement sleep. *Neuron, 29,* 145–156.

Lu, W. Y., Man, H. Y., Ju, W., Trimble, W. S., & Wang, Y. T. (2001). Activation of synaptic NMDA receptors induces membrane insertion of new AMPA receptors and LTP in cultured hippocampal neurons. *Neuron, 29,* 243–254.

Ma, T. P. (1997). The basal ganglia. In D. E. Haines (Ed.), *Fundamental neuroscience* (pp. 363–378). Cambridge: Churchill Livingstone.

MacDonald III, A. W., Cohen, J. D., Stenger, V. W., & Carter, C. S. (2000). Dissociating the role of the dorsolateral prefrontal and anterior cingulate cortex in cognitive control. *Science, 288,* 1835–1838.

Mactutus, C., Riccio, D., & Ferek, J. (1979). Retrograde amnesia for old (reactivated) memory: some anomalous characteristics. *Science, 204*(4399), 1319–1320.

MacWhinney, B. (1997). Implicit and explicit processes: Commentary. *Studies in Second Language Acquisition, 19,* 277–281.

Malinow, R., Schulman, H., & Tsien, R. W. (1989). Inhibition of postsynaptic PKC or calcium-calmodulin-dependent protein kinase II blocks induction but not expression of LTP. *Science, 245*(4920), 862–865.

Marrocco, R. T., & Davidson, M. C. (1998). Neurochemistry of attention. In R. Parasuraman (Ed.), *The attentive brain* (pp. 95–122). Cambridge, MA: MIT Press.

Martin, A. (1999). Automatic activation of the medial temporal lobe during encoding: Lateralized influences of meaning and novelty. *Hippocampus, 9,* 62–70.

Martin, A., & Chao, L. (2001). Semantic memory and the brain: structure and processes. *Current Opinion in Neurobiology, 11,* 194–201.

Martin, A., Wiggs, C. L., Ungerleider, L. G., & Haxby, J. V. (1996). Neural correlates of category-specific knowledge. *Nature, 379,* 649–652.

Martinez, A., Anllo-Vento, L., Sereno, M. I., Frank, L. R., Buxton, R. B., Dubowitz, D. J., Wong, E. C., Hinrichs, H., Heinze, H. J., & Hillyard, S. A. (1999). Involvement of striate and extrastriate visual cortical areas in spatial attention. *Nature Neuroscience, 2*(4), 364–369.

Martinez, J. L. Jr., Barea-Rodriguez, E. J., & Derrik, B. E. (1998). Long-term potentiation, long-term depression, and learning. In J. Martinez & R. Kesner (Eds.), *Neurobiology of learning and memory* (pp. 211–246). San Diego, CA: Academic Press.

Matsumoto, N., Hanakawa, T., Maki, S., Kimura, M., & Graybiel, A. M. (1999). Nigrostriatal dopamine system in learning to perform sequential motor tasks in a predictive manner. *Journal of Neurophysiology, 82*(2), 978–998.

McClelland, J. L., McNaughton, B. L., & O'Reilly, R. C. (1995). Why are there complementary learning systems in the hippocampus and the neocortex: Insights from the successes and failures of connectionist models of learning and memory. *Psychological Review, 102,* 419–457.

McEachern, J. C., & Shaw, C. A. (1996). An alternative to the LTP orthodoxy: A plasticity-pathology continuum model. *Brain Research Reviews, 22*(1), 51–92.

McGaugh, J. (2000). Memory: A century of consolidation. *Science, 287,* 248–251.

McGaugh, J. L., Roozendaal, B., & Cahill, L. (2000). Modulation of memory storage by stress hormones and the amygdaloid complex. In M. S. Gazzaniga (Ed.), *The new cognitive neurosciences* (pp. 1081–1098). Cambridge, MA : MIT Press.

Milham, M. P., Bainch, M. T., Webb, A., Barad, V., Cohen, N. J., Wszalek, T., & Kramer, A. F. (2001). The relative involvement of anterior cingulate and prefrontal cortex in attentional control depends on nature of conflict. *Cognitive Brain Research, 12,* 467–473.

Miller, E. K. (2000). The prefrontal cortex and cognitive control. *Nature Reviews Neuroscience, 1,* 59–65.

Miller, G. (2000). *The mating mind: How sexual choice shaped the evolution of human nature.* New York: Doubleday.

Miller, R., & Matzel, L. (2000). Memory involves far more than "consolidation." *Nature: Neuroscience, 1,* 214–216.

Millin, P., Moody, E., & Riccio, D. (2000). Interpretations of retrograde amnesia: Old problems redux. *Nature: Neuroscience, 2,* 68–70.

Milner, P. (1999). *The autonomous brain: A neural theory of attention and learning.* Mahwah, NJ: Lawrence Earlbaum Associates.

Misanin, J., Miller, R., & Lewis, D. (1968). Retrograde amnesia produced by electroconvulsive shock after reactivation of a consolidated memory trace. *Science, 160*(3827), 554–555.

Mogenson, G. J., Brudzynski, S. M., Wu, M., Yang, C. R., & Yim, C. C. Y. (1993). From motivation to action: A review of dopaminergic regulation of limbic→nucleus accumbens→ventral pallidum→pedunclulopontine nucleus circuitries involved in limbic-motor integration. In P. W. Kalivas & C. D. Barnes (Eds.), *Limbic motor circuits and neuropsychiatry* (pp. 193–236). Boca Raton, FL: CRC Press.

Montague, P. R., Dayan, P., Pearson, C., & Sejnowski, T. J. (1995). Bee foraging in uncertain environments using predictive hebbian learning. *Nature, 337,* 725–728.

Moore, C. J., & Price, C. J. (1999). A functional neuroimaging study of the variables that generate category-specific object processing differences. *Brain, 112,* 943–962.

Moscovitch, M., Yaschyshyn, T., Ziegler, M., & Nadel, L. (1999). Remote episodic memory and retrograde amnesia: Was Endel Tulving right all along? *Memory, consciousness and the brain: The Tallinn Conference* (pp. 331–345). New York: Psychology Press.

Mueller, G. E., & Pilzecker, A. (1900). *Psychology, 1*(1).

Nadel, L. (1990). Varieties of spatial cognition: Psychobiological considerations. *Annals of the New York Academy of Sciences, 608,* 613–636.

Nadel, L., & Moscovitch, M. (1997). Memory consolidation retrograde amnesia and the hippocampal complex. *Current Opinion in Neurobiology, 7,* 217–227.

Nadel, L., & Moscovitch, M. (1998). Hippocampal contributions to cortical plasticity. *Neuropharmacology, 37,* 431–439.

Nadel, L., Samsonovich, A., Ryan, L., & Moscovitch, M. (2000). Multiple trace theory of human memory: Computational neuroimaging and neuropsychological results. *Hippocampus, 10,* 352–368.

Nadel, L., & Willner, J. (1980). Context and conditioning: A place for space. *Physiological Psychology, 8*(2), 218–228.

Nader, K., Schafe, G., & LeDoux, J. (2000a). Fear memories require protein synthesis in the amygdala for reconsolidation after retrieval. *Nature, 406,* 722–726.

Nader, K., Schafe, G., & LeDoux, J. (2000b). The labile nature of consolidation theory. *Nature: Neuroscience, 1,* 216–219.

Nakamura, K., Sakai, K., & Hikosaka, O. (1999). Effects of local inactivation of monkey medial frontal cortex in learning of sequential procedures. *Journal of Neurophysiology, 82,* 1063–1068. Cambridge, MA: MIT Press.

Nakayama, K., & Joseph, J. S. (1998). Attention, pattern recognition, and pop-out in visual search. In R. Parasuraman (Ed.), *The attentive brain* (pp. 279–298). Cambridge, MA: MIT Press.

Nestor, P. G., & O'Donnell, B. F. (1998). The mind adrift: Attentional dysregulation in schizophrenia. In R. Parasuraman (Ed.), *The attentive brain* (pp. 95–122). Cambridge, MA: MIT Press.

Neville, H., Mills, D., & Lawson, D. (1992). Fractionating language: Different neural subsystems with different sensitive periods. *Cerebral Cortex, 2*(3), 244–258.

Niebur, E., & Koch, C. (1998). Computational architectures for attention. In. R. Parasuraman (Ed.), *The attentive brain* (pp. 163–186). Cambridge, MA: MIT Press.

O'Dell, T. (1999). Long-Term Potentiation. In G. Fain (Ed.), *Molecular and cellular physiology of neurons* (pp. 476–507). Cambridge, MA: Harvard University Press.

Ojemann, G., & Whitaker, H. (1978). The bilingual brain. *Archives of Neurology, 35,* 409–412.

O'Malley, J. M., & Chamot, A. U. (1990). *Learning strategies in second language acquisition.* Cambridge, MA : Cambridge University Press.

O'Scalaidhe, S. P., Wilson, F. A. W., & Goldman-Rakic, P.S. (1999). Face-selective neurons during passive viewing and working memory performance of rhesus monkeys: Evidence for intrinsic specialization of neuronal coding. *Cerebral Cortex, 9*(5), 459–475.

Oxford, R. L. (1990). *Language learning strategies: What every teacher should know.* New York: Newbury House/Harper & Row.

Paradis, M. (1994). Neurolinguistic aspects of implicit and explicit memory: Implications for bilingualism and SLA. In N. C. Ellis (Ed.), *Implicit and explicit learning of languages* (pp. 393–419). London: Academic Press.

Paradis, M. (1997). The cognitive neuropsychology of bilingualism. *Tutorials in bilingualism: Psycholinguistic perspectives.* Mahwah, NJ: Lawrence Erlbaum Associates.

Paradis, M. (1998). Acquired aphasia in bilingual speakers. *Acquired aphasia* (pp. 531–549). New York: Academic Press.

Parasuraman, R. (1998). The attentive brain: Issues and prospects. In R. Parasuraman (Ed.), *The attentive brain* (pp. 95–122). Cambridge, MA: MIT Press.

Paré, D., Collins, D. R., & Pelletier, J. G. (2002). Amygdala oscillations and the consolidation of emotional memories. *Trends in Cognitive Sciences, 6*(7), 306–314.

Parent, A. (1996). *Carpenter's human neuroanatomy.* Media, PA: Williams & Wilkins.

Pavlenko, A. (1999). New approaches to concepts in bilingual memory. *Bilingualism: Language and Cognition, 2*(3), 209–230.

Penfield, W., & Rasmussen, T. (1950). *The cerebral cortex of man: A clinical study of localization of function.* New York: Macmillan.

Perani, D., Cappa, S. F., Bettinardi, V., Bressi, S., Gorno-Tempini, M., Matarrese, M., & Fazio, F. (1995). Different neural systems for recognition of animals and man-made tools. *Neuroreport, 6,* 1637–1641.

Perani, D., Schnur, T., Tettamanti, M., Gorno-Tempini, M., Cappa, S. F., & Fazio, F. (1999). Word and picture matching: A PET study of semantic category affects. *Neuropsychologia, 37,* 293–306.

Pietres, A. (1895). Etude sur l'aphasie chez les polyglottes. *Revue De Medecine, 15,* 873–899. Translated in M. Paradis (Ed.), (1983). *Readings on aphasia in bilinguals and polyglots* (pp. 26–49). Montreal: Didier.

Plomin, R. (2001). The genetics of g in the human and mouse. *Nature Reviews Neuroscience, 2,* 136–141.

Posner, M. I., & Dahaene, S. (1994). Attentional networks. *Trends in Neuroscience, 17,* 75–79.

Posner, M. I., & DiGirolamo, G.J. (1998). Executive attention: Conflict, target detection, and cognitive control. In R. Parasuraman (Ed.) *The attentive brain.* Cambridge, MA: MIT Press.

Posner, M.I., & Petersen, S.E. (1990). The attention system of the human brain. *Annual Reviews Neuroscience, 13,* 25–42.

Potter, M., So, K., Von Eckardt, B., & Feldman, L. (1984). Lexical and conceptual representation in beginning and proficient bilinguals. *Journal of Verbal Learning and Verbal Behavior, 23*(1), 23–38.

Pryzbyslawski, J., & Sara, S. (1997). Reconsolidation of memory after its reactivation. *Behavioral Brain Research, 84,* 241–246.

Puce, A., Allison, T., Bentin, S., Gore, J. C., & McCarthy, G. (1998). Temporal cortex activation in humans viewing eye and mouth movements. *Journal of Neuroscience, 18,* 2188–2199.

Pulvermüller, F. (1992). Constituents of a neurological theory of language. *Concepts in Neuroscience, 3,* 157–200.

Pulvermüller, F. (1999). Words in the brain's language. *Behavioral & Brain Sciences, 22*(2), 253–336.

Pulvermüller, F., Haerle, M., & Hummel, F. (2000). Neurophysiological distinction of verb categories. *Neuroreport: For Rapid Communication of Neuroscience Research, 11*(12), 2789–2793.

Pulvermüller, F., Haerle, M., & Hummel, F. (2001). Walking or talking?: Behavioral and neurophysiological correlates of action verb processing. *Brain & Language, 78*(2), 143–168.

Pulvermüller, F., Lutzenberger, W., & Birbaumer, N. (1995). Electrocortical distinction of vocabulary types. *Electroencephalography & Clinical Neurophysiology, 94*(5), 357–370.

Pulvermüller, F., Lutzenberger, W., & Preissl, H. (1999). Nouns and verbs in the intact brain: Evidence from event-related potentials and high-frequency cortical responses. *Cerebral Cortex, 9*(5), 497–506.

Pulvermüller, F., & Mohr, B. (1996). The concept of transcortical cell assemblies: A key to the understanding of cortical lateralization and interhemispheric interaction. *Neuroscience & Biobehavioral Reviews, 20*(4), 557–566.

Pulvermüller, F., & Schumann, J. (1994). Neurobiological mechanisms of language acquisition. *Language Acquisition, 44,* 681–734.

Purves, D. (1997). Modulation of movement by the basal ganglia and cerebellum. In D. Purves, G. J. Augustine, D. Fitzpatrick, L. C. Katz, A. S. Lamantia, & J. O. McNamara (Eds.), *Neuroscience* (pp. 329–359). Sunderland, MA: Sinauer Associates.

Quartz, S. R., & Sejnowski, T. J. (1997). The neural basis of cognitive development: A constructivist manifesto. *Behavioral and Brain Sciences, 20,* 537–596.

Rand, M. K., Hikosaka, O., Miyachi, S., Lu, X., & Miyashita, K. (1998). Characteristics of a long-term procedural skill in the monkey. *Experimental Brain Research, 118,* 293–297.

Rempel-Clower, N., Zola, S., Squire, L., & Amaral, D. (1996). Three cases of enduring memory impairment after bilateral damage limited to the hippocampal formation. *Journal of Neuroscience, 16*(16), 5233–5255.

Ribot, T. (1881). *Les maladies de la memoire.* Paris: G. Bailliere.

Ridley, M. (2000). *Genome: The autobiography of a species in 23 chapters.* New York: Perennial.

Robbins, T. W. (1998). Arousal and attention: Psychopharmacological and neuropsychological studies in experimental animals. In R. Parasuraman (Ed.), *The attentive brain* (pp. 95–122). Cambridge, MA: MIT Press.

Robbins, T. W., & Everitt, B. J. (1996). Neurobehavioral mechanisms of reward and motivation. *Current Opinion in Neurobiology, 6,* 228–236.

Rolls, E. T. (1999). *The brain and emotion.* Oxford: Oxford University Press.

Rolls, E. (2000). Hippocampal-cortical and cortico-cortical backprojections. *Hippocampus, 10,* 380–388.

Romanski, L. M., Tian, B., Fritz, J. M. M., Goldman-Rakic, P. S., & Rauschecker, J. P. (1999). Dual streams of auditory afferents target multiple domains in the primate prefrontal cortex. *Nature Neuroscience, 2*(12), 1131–1136.

Rushworth, M. F. S., Krams, M., & Passingham, R. E. (2001). The attentional role of the left parietal cortex: the distinct lateralization and localization of motor attention in the human brain. *Journal of Cognitive Neuroscience, 13*(5), 698–710.

Rushworth, M. F. S., Paus, T., & Sipila, P. K. (2001). Attention systems and the organizations of the human parietal cortex. *The Journal of Neuroscience, 27*(14), 5265–5271.

Russell, W., & Nathan, P. (1946). Traumatic amnesia. *Brain, 69,* 280–300.

Ryan, L., Nadel, L., Keil, T., Putnam, K., Schayer, D., Troward, T., & Moscovitch, M. (2000). Hippocampal activation during retrieval of remote memories. *Neuro Image, 11,* 5396.

Sakai, K., Hikosaka, O., Miyauchi, S., Sasaki, Y., & Putz, B. (1998). Transition of brain activation from frontal to parietal areas in visuomotor sequence learning. *The Journal of Neuroscience, 18*(5), 1827–1840.

Sakai, K., Hikosaka, O., Takino, R., Miyauchi, S., Nielsen, M., & Tamada, T. (2000). What and when: Parallel and convergent processing in motor control. *Journal of Neuroscience, 20*(7), 2691–2700.

Saykin, A. J., Johnson, S. C., Flashman, L. A., McAllister, T. W., Sparling, M. B., Darcey, T. M., Moritz, C. H., Guerin, S. J., Weaver, J., & Mamourian, A. (1999). Functional differentiation of medial temporal and frontal regions involved in processing novel and familiar words: An fMRI study. *Brain, 122,* 1963–1971.

Scarr, S. (1996). How people make their own environments: Implications for parents and policy makers. *Psychology Public Policy, and Law, 2,* 204–228.

Scarr, S. & McCarthy, K. (1983). How people make their own environments: A theory of genotype→environment effects. *Child Development, 54,* 424–435.

Scherer, K. R. (1984). Emotion as a multi-component process: A model and some cross-cultural data. In P. Sharer (Ed.), *Review of personality and social psychology: Vol. 5. Emotions, relationships and health* (pp. 37–63). Beverly Hills, CA: Sage.

Schmidt, R. (1995). *Attention and awareness in foreign language learning.* Second Language Teaching and Curriculum Center: University of Hawaii at Manoa.

Schmidt, R., Boraie; D., & Kassabgy, O. (1996). Foreign language motivation: Internal structure and external connections. In R. L Oxford (Ed.), *Language learning motivation : Pathways to the new century* (pp. 13–87). University of Hawaii at Manoa: Second Language Teaching & Curriculum Center.

Schmidt, R., & Savage, W. (1992). Challenge, skill, and motivation. *PASAA, 22,* 14–28.

Schultz, W. (1997). Dopamine neurons and their role in reward mechanisms. *Current Opinion in Neurobiology, 7,* 191–197.

Schultz, W., Dayan, P., & Montague, P. R. (1997). A neural substrate of predicton and reward. *Science, 275,* 1593–1599.

Schultz, W., Romo, R., Ljungberg, T., Mirenowicz, J., Hollerman, J. R., & Dickinson, A. (1995). Reward-related signals carried by dopamine neurons. In J. C. Houk, J. L. Davis, & D. G. Bieser (Eds.), *Models of information processing in the basal ganglia* (pp. 233–248). Cambridge, MA: MIT Press.

Schumann, J. (1994). Where is cognition? Emotion and cognition in second language acquisition. *Studies in Second Language Acquisition, 16,* 231–242.

Schumann, J. H. (1990). Extending the scope of the acculturation/pidginization model to include cognition. *TESOL Quarterly, 24,* 667–684.

Schumann, J. H. (1997). *The neurobiology of affect in language.* Malden, MA: Blackwell. (Also published by the journal, *Language Learning,* as a supplement to volume *48,* 1997.)

Schumann, J. H. (2001a). Learning as foraging. In Z. Dörnyei & R. Schmidt (Eds.), *Motivation and second language acquisition* (pp. 21–28). Honolulu, HI: The University of Hawaii, Second Language Teaching and Curriculum Center.

Schumann, J. H. (2001b). Appraisal psychology, neurobiology, and language. In M. McGroarty (Ed.), *The Annual Review of Applied Linguistics (Vol. 21): Language and psychology* (pp. 23–42). New York: Cambridge University Press.

Scoville, W. B., & Milner, B. (1957). Loss of recent memory after bilateral hippocampal lesions. *Journal of Neurology, Neurosurgery and Psychiatry, 20,* 11–21.

Segal, N. L. (1999). *Entwined lives: Twins and what they tell us about human behavior.* New York: Dutton.

Selinker, L., & Selinker, P. (1972). *An annotated bibliography of U.S. Ph.D. dissertations in contrastive linguistics.* Washington, DC: Center for Applied Linguistics.

Shallice, T., Fletcher, P., Frith, C. D., Grasby, P., Frackowiak, R. S. J., & Dolan, R. J. (1994). Brain regions associated with acquisition and retrieval of verbal episodic memory. *Nature, 368,* 633–635.

Shors, T. J., & Matzel, L. D. (1997). Long-term potentiation: What's learning got to do with it? *Behavioral & Brain Sciences, 20*(4), 597–655.

Siapas, A. G., & Wilson, M. A. (1998). Coordinated interactions between hippocampal ripples and cortical spindles during slow wave sleep. *Neuron, 21,* 1123–1128.

Silva, A. J., & Giese, K. P. (1998). Gene targeting: A novel window into the biology of learning and memory. In J. Martinez, & R. Kesner (Eds.), *Neurobiology of Learning and Memory* (pp. 89–142). San Diego, CA: Academic Press.

Silva, A. J., Smith, A. M., & Giese, K. P. (1997). Gene targeting and the biology of learning and memory. *Annual Review of Genetics, 31,* 527–546.

Sinclair, J. M. (1991). *Corpus, concordance, and collocation.* Oxford: Oxford University Press.

Skehan, P. (1998). *A cognitive approach to language learning.* Honk Kong: Oxford University Press.

Skehan, P. (1989). *Individual differences in second-language learning.* London: Edward Arnold.

Skinner, R. D., & Garcia-Rill, E. (1993). Mesolimbic interactions with mesopontine modulation of locomotion. In P. W. Kalivas & C. D. Barnes (Eds.), *Limbic motor circuits and neuropsychiatry* (pp. 155–191). Boca Raton, FL: CRC Press.

Small, S. A., Nava, A. S., Perera, G. M., DeLaPaz, R., Mayeux, R., & Stern, Y. (2001). Circuit mechanisms underlying memory encoding and retrieval in the long axix of the hippocampal formation. *Nature Neuroscience, 4,* 442–449.

Smith, M. (1997). How do bilinguals access lexical information? *Tutorials in bilinguals: Psycholinguistic perspectives* (pp. 145–168). Mahwah, NJ: Lawrence Erlbaum Associates.

Sonnenstuhl, I., Eisenbeiss, S., & Clahsen, H. (1999). Morphological priming in the German mental lexicon. *Cognition, 72,* 203–236.

Sorra, K. E., & Harris, K. M. (2000). Overview on the structure, composition, function, development, and plasticity of hippocampal dendritic spines. *Hippocampus, 10,* 501–511.

Squire, L. R. (1992). Memory and the hippocampus: a synthesis from findings with rats, monkeys, and humans. *Psychological Review, 99,* 195–231.

Squire, L. R., & Alvarez, P. (1995). Retrograde amnesia and memory consolidation: a neurobiological perspective. *Current Opinion in Neurobiology, 5,* 169–177.

Squire, L., & Kandel, E. (1999). *Memory: From mind to molecules.* New York: Scientific American Library.

Squire, L. R., Knowlton, B., & Musen, G. (1993). The structure and organization of memory. *Annual Review of Psychology, 44,* 453–495.

Squire, L. R., & Zola-Morgan, S. (1991). The medial temporal lobe system. *Science, 253*(5026), 1380–1386.

Steinglass, M. (2001, September 2). An unlikely prodigy in an African new world. *New York Times, Section 2,* pp. 1, 20.

Sternberg, R. J. (1985). *Beyond IQ: A triarchic theory of human intelligence.* Cambridge, MA: Cambridge University Press.

Stolerman, I. P. (1993). Components of drug dependence: Reinforcement, discrimination and adaptation. *Biochemical Society (Great Britain) Symposium, 59,* 1–12.

Tannen, D. (1989). *Talking voices: Repetition, dialogue and imagery in conversational discourse.* Cambridge, MA: Cambridge University press.

Turving, E. (1972). Episodic and semantic memory. In E. Turving & W. Donaldson (Eds.), *Organization of memory* (pp. 381–403). New York: Academic Press.

Ullman, M. (2001a). The neural basis of lexicon and grammar in first and second language: the declarative/procedural model. *Bilingualism: Language and Cognition, 4*(1), 105–122.

Ullman, M. (2001b). A neurocognitive perspective on language: The declarative/procedural model. *Nature Reviews, 2,* 717–726.

Ullman, M. (2001c). The declarative/procedural model of lexical and grammar. *Journal of Psycholinguistics Research, 30,* 37–69.

Ullman, M. T., Corkin, S., Coppola, M., Hickok, G., Growdon, J. H., Koroshetz, W. J., & Pinker, S. (1997). A neural dissociation within language: Evidence that the mental dictionary is part of declarative memory, and that grammatical rules are processed by the procedural system. *Journal of Cognitive Neuroscience, 9,* 266–276.

Viskontas, I., McAndrews, M., & Moscovitch, M. (2000). Remote episodic memory deficits in patients with unilateral temporal lobe epilepsy and excisions. *Journal of Neuroscience, 20*(15), 5853–5857.

Volkmann, J., Hefter, H., & Lange, H. W. (1992). Impairment of temporal organization of speech in basal ganglia diseases. *Brain and Language, 43,* 386–399.

Wagner, A. D., Schacter, D. L., Rotte, M., Koustaal, W., Maril, A., Dale, A. M., Rosen, B. R., & Buckner, R. L. (1998). Building memories: Remembering and forgetting of verbal experiences as predicted by brain activity. *Science, 281,* 1188–1191.

Waksler, R. (1999). Cross-linguistic evidence for morphological representation in the mental lexicon. *Brain and Language, 68,* 68–74.

Warburton, D. M. (1991). The pleasures of nicotine. In F. Adlkofer & K. Thurau (Eds.), *Effects of nicotine on biological systems.* Berlin: Birkhauser Verlag.

Webster, M. J. & Ungerleider, L. G. (1998). Neuroanatomy of visual attention. In R. Parasuraman (Ed.), *The attentive brain* (95–122). Cambridge, MA: MIT Press.

Wienberger, N. (1995). Retuning the brain by fear conditioning. In M. Gazzaniga (Ed.), *The cognitive neurosciences* (pp. 1071–1089). Cambridge, MA: MIT Press.

Wilson, M. A., & McNaughton, B. L. (1994). Reactivation of hippocampal ensemble memories during sleep. *Science, 265,* 676–679.

Winner, E. (2000). Catching up with gifted kids. *Cerebrum, 3,* 37–54.

Wise, R. A. (1996). Neurobiology of addiction. *Current Opinion in Neurobiology, 6,* 243–251.

Witelson, S. F., Kigar, D. L., & Harvey, T. (1999). The exceptional brain of Albert Einstein. *The Lancet, 353,* 2149–2153.

Wood, P. L., & Altar, C. A. (1988). Dopamine release in vivo from nigrostriatal, mesolimbic and mesocortical neurons. *Pharmacological Reviews, 40,* 163.

Wood, P. L., & Richard, J. W. (1982). Morphine and nigrostriatal function in the rat and mouse: A role of nigral and striatal opiate receptors. *Neuropharmacology, 21,* 1305.

Wright, D., Loftus, E., & Hall, M. (2001). Now you see it; now you don't: Inhibiting the recall and recognition of scenes. *Applied Cognitive Psychology, 15,* 471–482.

Wu, Y. (2000). *The neurobiology of language acquisition.* Unpublished MA thesis, UCLA.

Zeki, S. (1993). *A vision of the brain.* London: Blackwell.

Zola-Morgan, S. M., & Squire, L. R.. (1990). The primate hippocampal formation: Evidence for a time-limited role in memory storage. *Science, 250*(4978), 288–290.

Author Index

Subject Index